DENTIST, n. A prestidigitator who, putting metal into your mouth, pulls coins out of your pocket.
—Ambrose Bierce, *The Devil's Dictionary.*

CONTENTS

PART ONE

THE TROUBLE WITH DENTISTS—INTRODUCING DR. POORWORK

PART TWO

WHAT EVERY PATIENT SHOULD KNOW

PART THREE

PART FOUR

PART FIVE

PART 1

THE TROUBLE WITH DENTISTS - INTRODUCING DR. POORWORK

When I first began the practice of dentistry it quickly struck me that the carefully planned, meticulously constructed restorations we had been taught to do in school were *not* characteristic of the dental work I saw in the mouths of the public. As time passed and I compared more and more examples of dentistry as actually practiced with dentistry as taught, I began to understand that an uncomfortably high percentage of dental work was substandard, much of it disgracefully so. Most distressing perhaps, was that the victims, without exception, never suspected that the dentistry they had received was anything less than the best; the American Dental Association's conspiracy of silence had done its job effectively.

It is shocking but true that a considerable number of dentists actually choose to do poor work. All bad dentists know how to practice good dentistry; all of them know how to make more money from bad dentistry than they ever could by doing good work; and all of them choose a high income in preference to their patients' health. Because these immoral dentists have so much in common, I have invented a single, typical dentist to represent the entire breed. I call him Dr. Poorwork. The villains of this book are all the Poorworks in the country, together with the dental societies, which are the machinery for the expression of Poorwork power.

For every dentist-hero in a white coat there may be one or more white-coated Poorworks leaning over victims in the dental chair. I say "there may be" because organized dentistry will not publish, and actually *suppresses,* all studies on the quality of dentistry as it is practiced. This book is a deliberate, angry exposé of bad dentistry and bad dentists. It is also intended to be a patient's handbook on dental practice. Armed with information, the reader will be better able to judge the quality of the dental care he and his family are receiving.

Bad dentistry, inadequate numbers of dentists and other trained dental personnel, public ignorance of the elements of dental care and oral hygiene, the efforts of the American Dental Association to suppress information badly needed by the public—these are some of the problems that have motivated the writing of this book. What can the nation do to turn the situation around? And what can any individual do, who simply wants reliable dental care for himself and his family? As a dentist, I should also like to ask, what must the dental profession itself do?

In this book I try to give the answer to some of these questions. I hope that this will help the average person understand just what it is that his dentist does for him, and what his dentist *should* do for him. And I hope that it will provide some remedies for the dental profession so that what is done and what should be done will be one and the same.

1

The Quality of
American Dentistry

A patient who walks into a dentist's office would be
shocked if he was told that there was a strong possibility, perhaps even a probability, that he was about to
undergo shamefully substandard dental treatment.
Yet it is a fact that the quality of dental service provided by different dentists varies from excellent to
almost unbelievably bad. Furthermore, it is difficult
to impossible for the *uninformed* layman to tell a good
dentist from a poor one. The difference is important.
A patient who receives good dental service has an
excellent chance of keeping his teeth and maintaining
good oral health indefinitely, while the patient who
receives poor dentistry has little chance of doing either.

Just how widespread is shoddy dentistry? It is unfortunate that there are no reliable statistics to guide
us. Since it has been the policy of the American Dental
Association to support the fiction that all dentists

5

maintain high standards of care, the lack of official statistics showing the true situation is understandable. I once heard of an investigation into the quality of dentistry in a certain area. This survey, sponsored by a local dental society, was dropped like a hot potato when some embarrassing results began to come in. A candid conversation with an honest dentist comes much closer to the true picture than the ADA fiction does. My own personal observations after fifteen years of practice are as follows:

1. *Of patients coming for initial examination, the great majority had dental restorations that were below state board licensing standards.*

2. *A high proportion of this poor work fell so far short of minimum standards as to be disgraceful. Patients with this type of care can usually look forward to frequent dental pain and, over the years, progressive loss of teeth.*

If a surgeon operates for an inflamed appendix, one expects him to do his job properly. He is not expected to leave the patient with probably future infection, possibly fatal. And yet a great many dentists routinely treat decayed teeth so that it is highly probable that their patients will later suffer infection and loss of teeth. The layman who seeks an easy explanation for so much slipshod dentistry may be amazed to learn that every licensed dentist in the country has demonstrated during his school training and in his state board examination that he is fully capable of practicing good dentistry. The following question is obvious, if its answer is not: If all dentists have been taught the necessary procedures and skills, and have proven their ability by earning a dental school degree and passing a state board examination, *how does one account for so much substandard dentistry?*

How indeed? It is a crucial question. The answer is at the core of the crisis facing dentistry today, and it suggests the extent of the crisis in the country's dental health tomorrow.

Before we develop the answer, let us first consider some of the requirements for an ordinary silver filling. In simplified terms, the following outline summarizes the major steps in the routine treatment of a back tooth with decay on a proximal (next-to-another) surface:

1. Complete removal of decay.
2. Removal of undermined tooth surface.
3. Proper extension of cavity form.
4. Insulation or lining, if deemed necessary.
5. Placement and condensation of the filling. (This involves the careful use and management of a matrix band and wedges.)
6. Marginal adaptation. (Very important, and occasionally very time-consuming.)
7. Restoration of the tooth to proper occlusion, form, and function.
8. Finishing and polishing.

These procedures must be done carefully and thoughtfully, *and they take time.* If complications arise—if the caries is extensive, if the pulp is involved, if any of dozens of difficulties arise—then these procedures take still longer. On a state board examination, the young dentists were given nearly three hours to complete just such a routine job, and the most accomplished men in the class took most or all of the time allowed because it took them that long to do a perfect job. I know of many dentists today, who in three hours, presume to stick in thirty such fillings.

Let us examine the consequences of a less-than-perfect job on our simple, two-surface filling discussed above. I will discuss each step in turn.

1. Complete removal of decay. Active decay left in a cavity will, over a period of time, spread like a cancer, progressively eating away the tooth until it can be saved only by elaborate and costly procedures. In a matter of months or years, a tooth improperly cleaned of decay will either be lost or, if the patient is lucky, it may be saved, though with great difficulty. Of the many sins committed by dentists, failure to remove decay is the most reprehensible. Yet there are many well-respected, prosperous dentists who *routinely* fail to remove decay from teeth because to do so would take too much time.

2. Removal of undermined tooth structure. This is that part of the tooth that has been weakened by loss of foundation tissue. It is, for example, sound tooth surface with its underpinnings decayed away. Areas thus weakened should be cut away before restoring the tooth. If this is not done, the weakened area is likely to chip or fracture away with use. Esthetically, teeth with translucent, off-color areas are often the result of failure to remove undermined enamel.

3. Proper extension of the cavity form. This is the preparation of the tooth to receive the filling; it involves considerations of both physics and physiology. The properties of the filling material dictate certain mechanical forms for the preparation. For example, there must be a sufficient mass cut from the tooth to allow for enough bulk of filling material for the filling to develop adequate strength. Broken fillings are often a result of inadequate bulk of filling material at

critical areas. From the physiological point of view, the preparation must extend to all areas of the tooth which are prone to decay in the future. This principle, known to dentists as "extension for prevention," is one of the oldest tenets of sound dentistry. Failure to observe this principle considerably increases the chance of recurrent decay around the filling.

4. Insulation or lining. This refers to the placement of a nonconductive, nontoxic material over the deepest and presumably most sensitive area of the prepared tooth prior to placing the filling. Lining reduces thermal and mechanical shock to the pulp.

5. Placement and condensation of the filling. In a typical two-surface filling, a matrix band must be placed around the tooth to serve as a mold for the condensation, or plugging, of the silver amalgam. There are several band techniques in use today which give satisfactory results; all must be handled carefully. The band should be wedged against the tooth beneath the gum level to help provide for flush margins between tooth and filling. Care must be taken to assure that the tooth remains completely dry and clean while being filled. Even the slightest amount of moisture contaminating the amalgam during placement will substantially weaken the completed filling. The amalgam must be firmly condensed, or packed, against the walls and floors of the preparation, and on the margins. The excess mercury component of the amalgam tends to rise to the surface. The soft, mercury-rich amalgam at the surface must be removed and the filling overpacked with fresh amalgam, which must then be very well packed. Finally the band

is removed and the filling is evened to the proper size with instruments called "carvers."

6. Marginal adaptation is a critical yet all-too-often-neglected task; perhaps half the fillings I see when examining new patients' mouths have bad margins. All margins of a filling must be finished flush with the tooth. If the filling is overextended, it must be trimmed, or the filling must be redone. A bad margin can destroy the soft tissue and bone support around a tooth, serve to catch and trap food, and lead to root decay.

7. Restoration of the tooth to proper occlusion, form, and function is accomplished with carving instruments. The bite is checked and rechecked and adapted until it is perfect. The filling is shaped to conform to proper anatomical size and shape for best function. Contacts with other teeth are restored and shaped until the tooth looks like a tooth again, and not merely a shapeless glob of silver amalgam.

8. At some later time, when the patient is next in the office and the filling has developed its full hardness, the filling is inspected and the amalgam carefully trimmed and polished as necessary.

It should be clear by now that the "simple filling" of a moderately decayed tooth is a complicated procedure. The slightest inattention to any detail will result in a substandard filling, one that has much less chance of ultimate success, one that should not be in your mouth or anybody's mouth. Yet there are dentists who do not pay enough attention to any of the above steps. These dentists, who for all we know may comprise even a majority of American dentists, are a disgrace to the dental profession, which so far has done nothing about them. Organized dentistry, in fact, has created a climate in which the substandard dentist not only exists but prospers, to the detriment of society and of all conscientious dentists. The situation is now assuming such scandalous proportions that it cannot exist much longer without causing an upheaval in the profession.

The central reason for the existence of bad dentistry is economic. Dentists, like practically everyone else, want to earn money. A dentist's income comes from his patients. If he has patients, he has income. Without them, he has no income. Let us suppose that you live in a working-class neighborhood of apartments and private homes, and that you are looking for a dentist. You hear there are two dentists, who have offices across the street from each other. By inquiring, you have discovered the information shown in the accompanying table. Based on this information, which is all you can get, to which dentist will you entrust your teeth?

Dr. Poorwork	*Dr. Goodwork*
1. Charges less.	1. Charges more.
2. Takes ten minutes.	2. Have to sit with mouth open for almost an hour.
3. Doesn't hurt.	3. Some types of work may cause discomfort.
4. Doesn't use a needle.	4. Has to use the needle.
5. Must be good; waiting room is always full.	5. Waiting room always empty.

But there are other, more important facts about our two neighborhood dentists. The patients of Dr.

Poorwork usually have trouble with their teeth and eventually they lose them, while the patients of Dr. Goodwork have relatively trouble-free mouths and keep their teeth. And over the years an individual patient of Dr. Poorwork pays a great deal more in dental fees as he loses his teeth than does an individual patient of Dr. Goodwork as he keeps his teeth — despite the fact that Dr. Goodwork "charges more" than Dr. Poorwork. One would think that these further facts about our two dentists might affect your decision about the choice of a dentist. And so they would, *if you knew them.* But there is no way for you to know, because Dr. Poorwork will certainly not tell you and, under the Code of Ethics of organized dentistry, Dr. Goodwork is not permitted to. There are some legitimate reasons for this restriction, but its total effect has been to perpetuate practices like those of Dr. Poorwork. Under this code Dr. Goodwork may say that his own work is good, but he is not allowed even to hint that Dr. Poorwork's dentistry is substandard. Who can blame the patient if he therefore concludes that the two dentists are equally competent and conscientious, and decides to avoid what he thinks is the extra inconvenience and expense of going to Goodwork? Perhaps, by counting his teeth twenty years later, the patient may eventually come to realize that Poorwork is destroying his mouth, but by this time most of the damage will have been done.

It is interesting to speculate about what will eventually become of Drs. Poorwork and Goodwork. Poorwork, as we are beginning to see, will make a fortune by destroying mouths. Goodwork, if he is lucky, may be able to settle for a modest income where he is now, accepting such patients as come to him; or he may leave the neighborhood in search of a Park Avenue practice; or else, as often happens, he may finally succumb to the pressures that produced Dr. Poorwork and become a Poorwork himself, in order to make a living.

It can be terribly frustrating for a dentist to try to maintain a high standard of work in the face of this situation. Here, by way of example, is an encounter typical of those I myself have had with prospective patients while trying to establish my practice:

A man, new to the neighborhood, presented himself for treatment. After a thorough examination, I found that he was in serious trouble. Many teeth were decayed. Nearly all his fillings had to be redone because of decay left underneath them, because of bad margins, and so forth. Missing teeth had to be replaced with expensive bridgework. He had gum problems which had been neglected. In short, he was a mess. Now the man was back in my chair, and I had to break the bad news to him. He was about to find out, from me, that he needed a lot of expensive work even though he had been receiving regular dental care all his life from Dr. Poorwork. Yet I had to be careful not to suggest that any of Poorwork's methods were at fault. Here is the way the interview went:

Me: "My examination discloses that you need to have a good deal of work. You should have periodontal therapy for your gums, you have extensive tooth decay, and your missing teeth should be replaced with fixed bridgework. These X-rays, models, and diagrams will show you why all this must be done and what will happen if it is not."

Patient *(interrupting):* "Wait a second. Why didn't my previous dentist tell me all this?"

Me: "As I was saying, this model will demon-the consequences of not replacing that tooth. As you see, this tooth will tip over and . . . "

Patient *(loudly):* "Why didn't Dr. Poorwork tell me this?"

Me: I don't know. "Now as this tooth tips over, the other . . .

Patient *(pointing):* How about this tooth here, Doc? It bothers me."

Me: "Here is an X-ray of that tooth. The dark area is decay. We will have to clean it all out and fix the tooth."

Patient: "But it was just filled two months ago!"

Me: "This tooth has to be fixed. The decay has to be removed. If the decay is not removed, a pulpal infection and abscess will result, as you can see on this diagram." *(I had to be careful. I couldn't use words like "refilled," or "done over"; they would have implied that Dr. Poorwork did poor work.)*

Patient: "Where did all this decay come from? The tooth was just filled."

Me: "I don't know. This diagram will show you . . . " Patient: "All you can say is, 'I don't know.' Sounds like you don't know anything."

Me *(losing patience):* "If a new filling is not made for that tooth . . . *(Now I realized I was in trouble. I had said "new filling," clearly hinting that the old one was no good. If word of this ever got back to Dr. Poorwork, he could have had me up before the Ethics Committee. I calmed down and tried to placate the patient.)* "Well, look. All I'm able to tell you is the results of the examination. Here is the present condition of your mouth, and there are my recommendations for treatment of your conditions."

Patient: "O.K., Doc. Tell me, what is this going to cost?"

I told him. It was a large sum, though a minimal fee for the work. The color drained from his face. As he slowly recovered he made his final speech. It was garbled and passionate, but words and phrases such as "high pressure sales talk," "crook," and so on, conveyed a clear impression of its meaning. He left, and I envisioned him on his way back to Dr. Poorwork, who would attend to this poor man's painful journey to full dentures, which I estimated were not far in his future. Too bad! I was new in the neighborhood and he might have been a source of referrals to help my practice. But as it was, I could be sure he wouldn't be much of a walking advertisement for me.

It is a pernicious fact that some types of dentistry in the average practice are much more lucrative than others. As a result, there is an economic factor present which can have a bearing on the diagnosis, the degree of the effect being related to the morality of the practitioner. Shall the dentist do procedure A for his patient when he can make twice the money by doing procedure B? Of course, a dentist of high moral standards has no difficulty with this problem. He strongly recommends what is best for the patient, without regard to his own financial well-being. But how about the thousands of Poorworks, who are interested only in income? As we shall see later on, this question will become even more pressing with the growth of social programs such as Medicaid.

Let us take a specific case. Prosthetic procedures, which involve the replacement of teeth, are much more lucrative than fillings. Why should Dr. Poorwork work hard to fill a tooth, when it is so easy to extract it and then collect a lush fee for replacing it? This reasoning is irresistable to many dentists. And why should Poorwork spend a lot of time filling a tooth perfectly, when the patient will pay him little for it? If the tooth is filled quickly and badly, he'll be paid just as much. Then there will be another job to be done on that same tooth in a few more years, then another, and then an extraction, and then a replacement—all at a fee. If the tooth is filled properly the first time, however, none of this subsequent work will be necessary, and none of the subsequent fees will be forthcoming. If the economic motive is paramount in man, how can we hope to have good dentistry so long as bad work is so much more lucrative than good work and bad dentists are so well protected by the ethical code?

Organized dentistry's public position is that of its Code of Ethics: All dentists do good work; therefore there cannot be any problem of quality, and any dentist who publicly says otherwise is violating the Code and is subject to discipline. But new problems are arising now that third parties, such as Medicaid, private and union insurance programs, and so on, are becoming increasingly involved in the provision of dental care. These third parties are slowly learning about the differences in the quality of dental work, and are at last beginning to make efforts to ensure that their funds are not spent on shoddy work. Organized dentistry has not been able to ignore this development. For example, a recent position paper written by a member of the New York State Dental Society's Board of Governors states that dentistry has failed, for many reasons, such as legal and *ethical* considerations, to protect the public from the *"very small percentage* of dentists" who do not routinely keep the quality of their work high. (Italics mine.) An editorial in a local dental society bulletin congratulates the writer of the paper for "his incisive description of the real problem."

This is one of the first examples I have seen of official recognition that a problem exists. The tactful and cautious phrase "very small percentage," in reference to low-quality dentists, is of particular interest. If Poorwork-style dentistry were confined to only a very small percentage of dentists there would be no need for position papers or editorial consternation. If Poorwork represented such a minute percentage, the contrast between his methods and those of legitimate dentistry would be easily discernible. In fact, there would be no problem. Today's problem exists only because Poorwork probably represents, rather than a very small percentage, a majority of dentists.

2

The Code of Ethics Versus the Morality of Dentists

Some years ago I tried to get my local dental society to look into the quality of dental work. While drumming up support for the move among my fellow dentists, I told one prominent dentist about an experience I had had with a man who had a tooth that had been badly treated, a mass of decay having been left in it by his regular dentist. Now the decay had progressed so far that the man had an acutely painful toothache, and he needed my help; his own dentist was unavailable. I am sure that his regular dentist's solution to this problem would have been to extract the tooth.

But this was not my way. After laboring an hour, I was confident the tooth was now in condition to be saved, and I quoted the man a fee. Far from being grateful, he objected violently, saying his dentist never took so long, never made him take an injection, and never charged any more for a permanent filling than

18

I proposed to charge for a temporary. My only defense would have been to tell him that his dentist had abused the tooth by leaving the decay in it, and that if the dentist had done his work well, by giving the job the time it needed, the toothache would never have occurred and the tooth would not be in jeopardy. Of course, I said no such thing, because I was mindful of the consequences to me of such a breach of so-called ethics. Dentists are not allowed to tell on one another.

I had told this story to the prominent man to try to get his help for my cause, which was in fact an attempt to get organized dentistry to come to grips with the problems of shoddy dentistry and the morality of dentists. When he had heard the tale, this dentist put his arm consolingly on my shoulder and said, in a fatherly way, "Sometimes you must do what is best for yourself, not what is best for the patient." I suppose that, as a young practitioner, I was expected to be grateful for this helpful advice. Perhaps I should have been, because the advice did at least give me an early insight into the morality of the dental profession. But it was not my first insight.

Some years earlier, as an undergraduate dental student, I had asked the dentist in charge of a clinic class why the course emphasized a rather esoteric treatment for restoring children's teeth in cases which, it seemed to me, would be better and more easily treated by conventional fillings. In answer, the instructor told me that the suggested treatment was more expensive and more lucrative. I asked if this justified its use. The dentist's reply summarized his morality in a succinct, unforgettable phrase. "We are not altruists," he said. I told him I thought that, as doctors, we were supposed to be altruists. "Come on, let's be honest about this," he replied. Evidently he believed a man is honest as long as he admits his dishonesty.

This points up the moral dilemma that underlies most of the problems facing dentistry today. Is a man moral if he is candid with his colleagues, but does not extend his candor to the public? Is a man moral who is honest with his colleagues, but deliberately misleads his patients? It is a shocking fact that the Code of Ethics of the American Dental Association answers these questions affirmatively by defining ethics *in terms of behavior toward other dentists rather than toward the public.* To express morality only in this way is like saying there should be honor among thieves. Dentists, according to the Code of Ethics, must hang together lest they be hanged separately. Let us examine the evolution of this concept of morality.

Historically the arts of healing and magic have been closely allied, mystery and secrecy being the major ingredients of both. The healer was a man who had knowledge, abilities, and power which set him apart from the others. To enter the fraternity of the healers required privileged selection and periods of training and formal initiation, the initiate always being sworn to secrecy. Care was taken to maintain the mystery and the distance between healer and patient. To this end a mysterious new nomenclature was developed, and stringent requirements were established for the behavior of the patients. Elaborate rationalizations were prepared to explain away the failure of the healer's methods. (It was said, for example, that the healer *never* failed; instead, an evil spirit borne by the patient was at fault.) Any challenge to the supremacy of the healers was countered by mumbo-jumbo coupled with threats of supernatural retaliation. Such tactics were almost invariably effective. From such beginnings have today's healing arts sprung, and a modern observer might well say that they haven't sprung very far.

The medical and dental societies still have many trappings of the secret society; it has been their policy to prevent the public from acquiring any substantive knowledge of medical or dental practice. The dental society, for example, imposes a complete censorship on the public writings and utterances of its members. The rationale has been that laymen do not have the background to interpret professional information. In the hands of the public a little knowledge is a dangerous thing, and any hard facts may be misconstrued; much better that people be kept ignorant of these sensitive matters. As for the patients, they can rely on the benevolent condescension of us doctors; everything will be all right as long as nobody asks any questions.

And so prescriptions are still written in Latin, and doctors say "hemorrhage" instead of "bleeding" and "sequellae" instead of "consequences." Patients have been trained to suffer the rudest treatment without complaint. A patient with a seven-o'clock appointment may sit and wait over an hour at an office or hospital or clinic and not grumble; he would not put up with such discourtesy anywhere else. Before initiating any complex procedures, the doctor requires the signing of a release; he is never to be at fault no matter what the result. Curiously enough, the doctor cannot even be prosecuted for *intentional* malpractice, but only for accidental malpractice. (More on this later.) A patient's attempt to elicit information from the doctor usually meets with evasion. Questions receive stock answers or are greeted with an "I'm-too-busy" or "Don't-bother-yourself-about-that; leave-everything-to-us" attitude. Any answers are often less than completely truthful. For example, a patient who asks why work on his tooth cost fifteen dollars may be told that there were "three fillings in one tooth." A completely truthful answer would be that the dentist made only one filling, but that it was large and unusually time-consuming, and since the real basis of fees is time, the filling cost more. Such explanations are rarely given, for they invite the patient to try to understand the business aspect of the profession, and they reduce the knowledge and mystery gap between doctor and patient.

This gap is very much a part of modern practice. The greater it is, the more the power of the doctor over his patient and the less this power is likely to be questioned. The professions are very aware of this, and professional behavior in this respect actually amounts to collusion among doctors to maintain the general ignorance.

The Code of Ethics of the dental profession is a modern outgrowth of the doctor's ancient desire to keep his secrets from the public. In a copy of the Code published by a local dental society one looks in vain for any convincing emphasis that the dentist's first obligation is to his patient. The Code, as written, is simply a manual of business conduct applying to the behavior of dentists toward other dentists. The standards are intended to protect dentists from each other and to insulate the profession as a whole against any criticism or attempt to undermine the practitioner's *privileges*. His *responsibility* to serve the public is never emphasized.

Thus, in the Code of Ethics there are articles relating to advertising, office signs, taking patients from another dentist, hiring a hygienist with a following, volunteering one's name for a referral list which would publish fees, and so forth. Particular emphasis is given to strictures concerning any attempt to obtain new patients by criticizing the work of the patient's previous dentist. This concept has been enlarged to the point that a dentist may never say anything to a patient or the public that might be construed as criticism of a dentist or the profession as a whole. No dentist is even permitted to publish anything or make a speech about anything professional without first submitting the material to the society for approval. This censorship is absolute, and violators are subject to severe discipline by the society, which would be furious were any of its secrets given publicity.

The Code does not espouse the idea that the dentist should consider the public's welfare. The individual dentist, other dentists, and the profession as a whole come first. In fact, the public is considered *only* as a hostile force from which dentists must be protected. This protection is achieved by never permitting the public, even for a moment, to have access to information that might cause some unpleasant questions to be asked. Take, for example, a simple truth: A person who gives his mouth good care should never lose important teeth except, perhaps, in his later years.[1] This, in the light of modern achievements, is an unquestioned fact, agreed upon by good dentists everywhere. But the ADA does not want the public to know this established fact, because patients who take care of their teeth but lose them anyway might begin to question the quality of the work done by their dentists. And so an elemental truth about modern dentistry, that people should not lose teeth, is suppressed. As this is written, a dentist

---

[1] Of course there are exceptions. Impacted wisdom teeth do have to be removed in some cases, though these are not important teeth. Accidents and injury sometimes necessitate the removal of teeth. Very rarely, some other type of situation arises which frustrates the best preventive efforts of dentist and patient and results in the loss of an important tooth. But such instances are so very rare that I estimate that the statement, "A person who gives his mouth good care should never lose important teeth except, perhaps, in his later years," is applicable in ninety-nine per cent of all cases.

who recently made a public statement of this fact about teeth is being disciplined by his local dental society.

The ethical Code leads to some Alice-in-Wonderland results. Take the example of the moral dentist who spends a good amount of time properly filling one surface of a tooth, and charges five dollars, a common fee for a one-surface filling, and of the immoral dentist who makes three small pits in the tooth surface, charging fifteen dollars "for three fillings." In summary, the immoral dentist does an inferior job, knows that it is inferior, knows that the tooth is odds-on to give trouble in the future, and knows that it is the poorest treatment for the patient. He does the job the way he does it solely to make more money in less time. One might think that such behavior on the part of a professional man would be clearly unethical. Wrong! According to the remarkable Code of Ethics, what this immoral dentist does is completely ethical and not open to question. As long as he maintains that his treatment, obviously dreadful though it be, was *in his judgment* correct, then his conduct is beyond reproach. Now consider the conscientious dentist who spends triple the time properly restoring the tooth for one-third the fee. If he says that the three-pit filling in another tooth is bad work and should be replaced before it causes trouble, then, according to the Code, *he* is clearly unethical.

To say anything that might be construed as criticism of another dentist's work is unethical, but intentionally to destroy a patient's tooth for increased profit is absolutely ethical. Such is the prescribed Code of Ethics of dentistry.

It is easy to imagine the results of such a code. A dentist beguiled by the glitter of greatly increased income can too easily bring himself to say that in his judgment the three-pit filling is proper for the case, particularly when he knows that this judgment will never be questioned by the patient or by any other dentist. The result is the condition of dental practice in this country today, a condition that has made the average citizen feel that to lose teeth is inevitable despite dental care.

The Code's message to the dentist is clear: The dentist himself is the sole judge and final authority on ethical behavior toward his patient. This is, in effect, an invitation to the dentist to do what he will. If he decides to mutilate a patient's dentition because doing so will earn him a huge profit, that is his business; the official morality of dentistry is indifferent to such practices. Yet I recall being told that the Code is essentially the Golden Rule. Dentistry's paraphrase of the Golden Rule seems to be, Do unto others as you would have others do unto you only if these others are dentists. The public be damned!

According to the Code, *the only one qualified to make a moral judgment concerning work done for a patient is the very same dentist who is in a position to profit greatly from the destruction of the patient's dental health.*

Are there any legitimate reasons for such provisions in what is supposed to be a code of *ethics*? Here are the reasons commonly advanced in defense of the Code, with my comments:

> *If I criticize a dentist's work, the dentist may turn out to be my buddy across the street, or perhaps the patient's uncle. It will be embarrassing.* True enough, but my obligation should be to the health of the patient rather than the prevention of embarrassment. That the dentist is my buddy does not invest him with license to do immoral dentistry.
>
> *If I criticize someone else's work, then some other*

dentist will be free to criticize mine. True again, but my primary responsibility is to the patient's oral health and not to my own immunity from criticism.

If I make decisions concerning another dentist, what will happen when someone wants to make decisions about me? If another dentist is behaving immorally, a decision should be made to compel him to behave morally. I should have no objections to a ruling that I must behave fairly toward my patients.

Criticism of any phase of dentistry hurts us all; if one dentist gets a bad press, the entire profession suffers. This is the crux. The central criterion for moral judgment is *not* whether I or other dentists are going to be hurt, but whether I am prepared to do the right thing; yet the "ethical" Code is solely concerned with the selfish interests of the dentists. This use of the word ethical is most ironic.

It is unfair to criticize another man's work. I don't know the circumstances under which the job was done. The patient may have been gagging or even throwing a fit; such conditions may have made satisfactory work impossible. This argument, though universally heard, is nonsense. Inquiry among good dentists and the experience of my own practice has led me to believe that a satisfactory result can be obtained if the dentist is willing to spend the necessary time. I am hard pressed to think of an exception from my own practice. But the widespread use of this argument suggests that the practices of many dentists are composed entirely of epileptics continually throwing fits.

It is unfair to criticize another dentist, because it is impossible to judge the quality of dental work. This commonly heard argument is also nonsense. A thorough clinical and X-ray examination will almost invariably expose poor dental work.

In summary, the Code of Ethics simply mediates the business dealings of dentists to one another, and is set up to further the convenience, privilege, mutual advantage, and profit of dentists. Its major function is to guard the right of dentists to be the sole judge of what they do, and to uphold their practice of doing whatever they please without risk of outside interference.

But can it be true that dentists operate under no effective restraint? How about the laws concerning malpractice? Legally, malpractice is injurious treatment contrary to accepted rules. The rub is that if a dentist decides to fill a tooth without removing decay, there is nobody who can prove that the procedure was contrary to accepted rules, because each dentist is free to establish his own rules according to the convenient dictates of his "judgment." But if inferior treatment rendered simply for the larger profit to the dentist were called malpractice, as it is in common usage, then I would say that I have seen thousands of products of dental malpractice in people's mouths. From the point of view of the law, nevertheless, there was no malpractice, since all this dentistry was done according to accepted rules. Yet malpractice judgments *are* granted against dentists. These judgments are nearly always given for the results of accidents. If a dentist accidentally dropped an instrument down the throat of a patient, or cut his cheek with a drill, this might amount to legal malpractice. But from a moral point of view any such accidental injury is *unintentional* and therefore guilt-free, not deliberate or for the profit of the dentist. It is only *intentional* malpractice that goes unchecked and unpunished. According to legal precedent, however, intentional, *knowing* malpractice of the sort Dr. Poorwork perpetrates daily calls for a judgment of *punitive* damages. I recently read of a case in which a patient was awarded a substantial sum because his dentist did not perform needed periodontal work. Will this be the first in a series of legal reprisals against Dr. Poorwork?

The time has come for change; the gap between dentist and patient is an intolerable relic of the past. People should by now have learned to respect the dentist because of his knowledge, capability, and legitimate accomplishments, and not because of his distance, arrogance, or contrived aura of mystery. The past performance of dentists does not suggest that they deserve to continue to be their own judges. If the healing professions do not soon demonstrate that they are capable of maintaining a high standard of moral conduct, then the public will certainly decide to intervene. Too much is at stake to allow the present moral climate to continue.

In dentistry, the whole future performance of the profession may be at stake. Consider for example, the career alternatives available to today's new dental graduate. Upon investigation, he finds the following avenues open to him:

1. In some cities he can go into work in as an employee in a high-volume, high-speed, low-quality Medicaid practice, earning up to $200 a day to start. In time he can become a partner in his own Medicaid practice, with annual earnings in six figures.
2. He can go into a high-volume, high-speed, low-quality city neighborhood practice, possibly including some Medicaid work, and be satisfied, after a few years, with an income of thirty to fifty thousand a year.
3. He can consider a high-volume, high-speed, low-quality suburban practice, with little or no

Medicaid, but with prospects of excellent income.

4. He can open a high-quality, very-high-fee practice in a luxury area, and hope for an excellent income only after years of building the practice. At least with a so-called Park Avenue practice, he will have an opportunity really to help the people he treats.

5. He can try to establish a high-quality, medium-fee, neighborhood practice. Here he will have to be satisfied with an income that will be adequate but modest by the standards of the above practices; even this adequate income will not be realized for some time.

Faced with these alternatives, and guided by the present standards of morality in the profession, in which direction will the new dentist turn? In order to give the good service for which he has been trained, he will have to choose between a Park Avenue practice, so difficult to establish, and the much less rewarding prospect of a good-quality neighborhood practice. Yet Park Avenue dentistry cannot be the ultimate answer for a man who believes it is not only the wealthy who deserve good care, and the difficulties of neighborhood practice may prove to be too much even for the well intentioned young dentist. Thus, unless something is done soon, the prevailing morality of the dental profession may push a whole new generation of dentists into the Poorwork tradition.

Our society is not so extravagant that it can afford to spawn another generation of Poorworks. Dental manpower is in such short supply that we must demand the maximum effectiveness from our dentists; Poorworks are wholly ineffective in treating dental disease. Particularly now, with the advent of newer social concepts and programs for the dissemination of treatment, it becomes more than ever urgent to maintain an effective standard of care. The moral climate in which the economic incentives operate to reward immoral and ineffective treatment more than moral and effective treatment must be altered. The system which provides the maximum economic incentive for slipshod dentistry, and which encourages dishonest treatment by rewarding it financially and by granting it immunity from criticism and from the law has failed in the past and will be disastrous in the future.

3

Why Good Dentists Turn Bad

The layman may be surprised to learn that good dentistry can be risky for the dentist. In many areas, nevertheless, dentists do consider it risky to try to do good work. To understand how this can be true, let us remember that, though some patients are well educated in the methods and objectives of good dentistry, such people are in the minority. The dental expectations of the less sophisticated, vast majority can be summed up as follows: They expect dentistry to relieve them of pain; they want it to be quick, painless, and cheap; and they don't want to be involved with postoperative pain or inconvenience. They have never understood that the major objective of dentistry is to maintain the health of the mouth and to save the teeth. Their experience with dentists has led them to conclude that dentistry consists of a series of palliative treatments while, over the years, the patient gradually loses his

31

teeth. After all, it's normal for most people to lose their teeth as they grow old, isn't it? The dentist's functions, to these people, are to relieve pain and to put in new teeth as they take out the old, "bad" teeth. It has not yet gotten through to the majority that *teeth should not be lost,* and that if cared-for teeth *are* lost, then something must be wrong with the dental work.

With this in mind, let us return to the idea that good dentistry is risky for the dentist. Suppose a dentist opens an office in a typical, mixed white-collar and working-class neighborhood. Our new dentist, young Dr. Goodwork, wants his new neighbors to become his patients. Time-honored economic practice dictates that Goodwork must supply demand, demand in this case being for quick, painless, and cheap work. He well realizes that if he lets the word get out that he will meet this demand, he may soon be blessed with a lively practice. But he is still young and idealistic, and he believes that he should be able to educate his patients to welcome good work. After all, he thinks, isn't good work much cheaper in the long run? Doesn't it involve, over the years, less pain and inconvenience? And doesn't it result in healthier mouths and bodies, and in keeping one's own teeth? Dr. Goodwork sets about to present his conception of good dentistry to his new patients. It is right here that he runs headlong into the first risk of good dentistry.

Risk Number One: The risk of being considered expensive.

Let us first assume that Dr. Goodwork has gotten a new patient to accept his fee for an examination. (The patient's prior dentist may or may not have used X-rays, and probably did not conduct thorough examinations.) If the former dentist was Poorwork, it is likely the patient's mouth will have to be thoroughly overhauled, and at a high cost. If he has few fillings, it is probable that he has a periodontal condition that was never properly treated and now needs attention, again at much higher fees than Poorwork charged for his variety of "cleaning." If the patient is young and needs relatively little work, he will still notice that Goodwork's fees are higher for what he imagines is similar work. (Remember that Goodwork is not permitted to imply that Poorwork's dentistry is anything but satisfactory.) In any case, the new patient is likely to be floored by the stated fee. After all, Dr. Poorwork never mentioned he needed *so much* work. So, from Dr. Goodwork's first contact with people in the neighborhood, the word spreads that he is expensive, even though his fees actually represent a spectacular bargain when compared on a time-and-result basis with those of Dr. Poorwork.

Risk Number Two: The risk of being considered a "conman."

Dr. Goodwork is frustrated in his efforts to justify his fees to his prospective patients. "Ethically," he is restricted to a dispassionate presentation of the existing condition, the need for correction, and the intended treatment. He can show charts, diagrams, slides, models, and movies; he can discuss dental theory at length; he can claim that what he intends to do will *save* money and teeth in the long run. But, asks the patient, isn't this exactly what his old dentist, Dr. Poorwork, has been doing all along, and at half the cost? Dr. Goodwork has a convincing answer to this critical question, but he is not permitted to give it. He knows that his own fee is higher because Poorwork does not take the time to do proper work. He knows that the patient's mouth has to be rehabilitated at high cost precisely because of Poorwork's cheap, shoddy dentistry. But the Code of Ethics seals his lips, and very often the would-be patient walks out unconvinced, spreading the word that Dr. Goodwork is a fast talker or a "conman, trying to sweet-talk people into a lot of work at high fees."

Risk Number Three: The risk that you will be accused of prescribing unnecessary work.

"If he doesn't see a hole, he'll make one." This statement is often made by laymen who suspect a dentist's honesty. Suppose a patient, after many years with busy Dr. Poorwork, decides to give young Dr. Goodwork a chance. Dr. Goodwork, upon examination, prescribes hundreds of dollars of work. Dr. Poorwork, just six months ago, hadn't mentioned anything like this. So the patient goes back to Poorwork, who shrugs his shoulders and says he doesn't see the need for all that work. Now the word spreads that Dr. Goodwork tries to generate business by prescribing unnecessary work.

Risk Number Four: The risk of being considered a painful dentist.

The word "dentistry" has always evoked the word "pain." The fear of pain has been enough to cause many people to avoid routine care, and a reputation for inflicting pain can be fatal to a practice. Nevertheless, compared with Dr. Poorwork's methods, some of Dr. Goodwork's procedures are going to produce discomfort, most often postoperatively. The periodontal curettage and scalings that Dr. Goodwork does in treating gum conditions usually leave the gums sore and tender for a few days; Dr. Poorwork's five-minute "cleanings" and chemical "gum treatments" never hurt anybody—not, anyway, until years later, when the teeth may loosen from periodontal disease. When Dr. Goodwork fills a tooth, he drills deeply enough to remove *all* decay and to prepare the tooth properly for the restoration. His deep fillings are occasionally sore for days afterwards, and may retain thermal sensitivity for up to a month. Dr. Poorwork's fillings, with a minimum of drilling and too often with much of the decay left in, rarely hurt postoperatively—until, perhaps, the tooth abscesses, which may not happen for years.

X-rays often show Dr. Goodwork a lot of decay that has been left under a filling made by Dr. Poorwork. Though the tooth still shows no symptoms, Dr. Goodwork knows that if he does not act at once it will soon require at least a costly root canal treatment, and that at worst it will be so badly rotted away that restoration will no longer be possible, and the tooth will have to be extracted. At this moment the tooth may be at the point where the decay is breaking through to the pulp, where a bacterial invasion will soon lead to an abscess. The sooner the tooth is worked upon, the better. Dr. Goodwork begins the arduous, difficult, delicate job of removing all decay and trying to avoid involvement of the pulp. This task, Dr. Goodwork ruefully observes, would have been easy when the filling was first done, before the decay had spread; but easy as the job would then have been, Dr. Poorwork did not take the additional time to do it properly.

This situation has many possible results. Suppose Dr. Goodwork is miraculously able to complete the work without a pulpal involvement, and that he places a well-made filling. The chances are that this tooth will be sensitive to hot and cold for several weeks. Later on the tooth may abscess anyway, because of the pulpal damage caused by the proximity of so much decay. If, while excavating the decay, Dr. Goodwork found that there *was* an involvement with the pulp, he might try a pulpotomy or a pulp-capping, simple endodontic procedures with good chances of success, instead of immediately instituting major root canal procedures, costly work which could be done later, if necessary. Sometimes the success of these procedures lies in the balance for months; sometimes they fail and root canal is necessary; in any case, the patient can expect some postoperative discomfort. Where does all this leave Dr. Goodwork in the eyes of his patient? Remember that Dr. Poorwork had filled this tooth quickly and easily and that the tooth had never hurt until Dr. Goodwork got his hands on it. The patient has to take a lot on faith if Dr. Goodwork tells him that what was done, pain included, was all for the best. Since he assumes that Poorwork also did the right thing for the tooth, the only decision he can reach is to stay clear of Dr. Goodwork from now on. The word goes out again: Dr. Goodwork spells pain and trouble.

Risk Number Five: The risk of being considered an inept amateur.

It is difficult for a patient to judge a dentist's ability. The patient in the previous paragraph might easily believe that Dr. Goodwork's skill is wanting. He takes longer to do a job and he sweats and strains and mutters to himself, and the patient experiences discomfort. The legendary criterion of "gentle hands" cannot be sympathetically applied by one who has been sitting in a chair, mouth open and face contorted, for an hour. But twenty years hence today's patient of Dr. Goodwork may adopt a better standard when he notices that he still has all his teeth, while his friends, still loyal to Dr. Poorwork, are missing many of theirs. Unfortunately, Dr. Goodwork, who has a family to support, may not find it possible to wait so long for people to appreciate him. And meanwhile the standard of competence is Dr. Poorwork, a man who is so skillful that he fills teeth quickly and painlessly. Should we be surprised, therefore, to learn that people are saying that Dr. Goodwork is clumsy and incompetent?

Is it risky to perform substandard dental work? No, not as long as people are conditioned to view the loss of teeth as a regular part of the aging process. Just as the bad surgeon buries his poor work, so Dr. Poorwork extracts his. The only risk he runs is that he will get into a high tax bracket.

PART 2

WHAT EVERY PATIENT SHOULD KNOW

4

On the Mouth

To understand some of the things said later in the book about the sorts of work a dentist does—or ought to do —it may be helpful to have a quick description of some of the basic facts about teeth and their treatment.

The mouth is an extraordinarily complex and vitally important part of the anatomy. Though the long list of all its particular divisions and all their exact tasks has no place here, it may nevertheless be useful to itemize certain strategic features and some of their functions.

The mouth contains the apparatus for evaluating and selecting fuel for the body; all the taste buds are here. The mouth includes the lips, the tongue, the cheeks, the teeth, and the muscles of mastication, which, taken together are the complete apparatus for manipulating, macerating, and swallowing food. Here, too, are the salivary glands, that manufacture a fluid with remarkable chemical and physiological properties, and here also we find a valvular apparatus that routes incoming food and air into the proper internal systems. We may recall, furthermore, that it is through the mouth that we whistle, speak, sing, and shout. Most people are aware that the mouth experiences temperatures ranging from the freezing point of iced desserts to the scalding heat of hot coffee, but how many know that in healthy people it regularly plays host to over eighty varieties of microorganisms? Because the mouth is exposed to air, it is continually being dried out; because the salivary glands are doing their job, it is continually being remoistened. The mouth often harbors various plastic and metallic compounds that are used as dental restorations; these compounds include metals of varying composition which, when bathed in the electrolytic saliva, produce electric current. I will forbear discussing the role assigned to the mouth in the development and expression of the psyche according to the Freudians.

The tongue is a strong, active muscle, which assists in the placement of food for chewing, in swallowing, and in the formation of words. Its strength is quite surprising. For example, if it habitually presses on one or more teeth, it can cause them to move. In swallowing and in speech, the efforts of the tongue are backed up by the muscles of the lips and cheek. The jaw muscles, or muscles of mastication, are very powerful; in the human body their strength is exceeded only by those of the calf. Using only the jaw muscles, for example, one can remove the cap from a bottle, break bones, and suspend oneself from the teeth, a la circus performers. (But don't try any of these stunts, please; you'll damage your teeth if you do.) On the inside of each cheek there is a small lump; these are the openings for the right and the left parotid salivary glands.

These normal structures sometimes frighten people who, never having noticed them before, suddenly see them for the first time and run to their dentists or physicians in fear that the lumps are cancerous. Other odd but normal structures are the torus palatinus, a symmetrical lump in the middle of the hard palate, and the torus mandibularis, two lumps, one on each half of the interior aspect of the lower jaw, which are symmetrical in that they look like mirror images of each other. Not everyone has a torus, but those who do can be assured that they are perfectly normal.

The most significant factor in the intra-oral environment is the saliva, which is produced by the salivary glands located in the cheeks and in the floor of the mouth. These glands discharge their output into the mouth through individual ducts. The saliva lubricates the food, making mastication and swallowing easier, and it helps in the digestion of starches. The normal output of the salivary glands is affected by emotional states as well as by hunger, the intake of food, and other stimuli. Fear or great stress causes discharge by the parotid salivary glands, in the cheeks. Parotid saliva is relatively thick and heavy. When animals or people who are tremendously angry or fearful foam at the mouth, they are displaying their parotid saliva. The other salivary glands, which produce a lighter secretion, respond to eating and to thoughts of eating.

The saliva is an extraordinary natural chemical buffer. It is able instantly to neutralize acids and bases; thus it protects the sensitive intra-oral tissue from damage. It is a natural disinfectant; ask any cat. An open wound on any body surface is likely to become infected if untreated, but not so in the mouth. Even the gaping hole in bone and tissues that is left by an extraction rarely gets infected, thanks to the protective action of the saliva. This is the more amazing in view of the huge population of microorganisms in the saliva, where over eighty known varieties of bacteria, fungi, filamentous forms, and so on, have been found to occur normally. Under conditions other than those in the mouth most of these would be capable of producing wicked infections. But in the environment of the saliva the organisms tend to balance each other off, and to stay under control, so that no harmful infection results. Yet the saliva may play a critical role in the development of tooth decay; this possibility will be discussed later.

The periodontium (peri = around; dont = tooth), which is the area immediately around the teeth, consists of what dentistry knows as the supporting structures of the teeth. Here are the jawbones, the periodontal ligaments, and the gums, or gingivae; it is these tissues that keep the teeth where they belong. Periodontal disease is, in effect, an impairment of the health of these supporting structures.

The periodontal ligament consists of a series of short fibers which attach the tooth to its socket in the bone, each fiber connecting with the bone at one end and the root of the tooth at the other. That part of each jawbone that immediately surrounds the teeth, and to which the periodontal ligaments anchor the teeth, is known as the alveolar bone, which has extraordinary properties compared to those of other types of bone. Pressure applied to the alveolar bone in certain directions results in resorption of the bone, with the bone elements decalcifying and being carried off by the circulatory system. On the other hand, pressure applied to the bone in other directions can cause it to grow stronger. As we shall see later on, it is these surprising properties of alveolar bone that make it possible for a child's dentition to erupt and develop normally. But these properties also explain the lateral movement of teeth that may occur if the space from which a tooth has been extracted is not promptly filled. Such tooth migration, as it is sometimes called, can lead to a "bad bite," or malocclusion, with the result that powerful biting pressures are concentrated in only one or two teeth in each jaw, instead of being spread evenly across all teeth. If the concentrated pressures that are passed on to the jawbone result in the resorption of the alveolar bone, as they often do, then the periodontal ligament will atrophy and the tooth will become loose; this is an important cause of periodontal disease. But though these properties of alveolar bone may be a source of grief to some, especially adults who receive poor dental care, they offer orthodontists a way to help youngsters with malposed teeth, which may cause a poor appearance, malocclusion, or both. By the use of braces, the orthodontist applies controlled pressures in carefully programmed steps so that the bone is resorbed in some areas and built up in others. The teeth then move in the direction of adjacent, controlled resorption and away from adjacent, controlled growth of alveolar bone. Thus they are slowly and securely maneuvered into the desired positions.

The teeth are layered, or laminated, organs, each of which is divided into two major anatomic parts: the root, or that part of the tooth which is beneath the gum and which is normally set into the jawbone, and the crown, which is the visible part of the tooth. Many people consider the crown to be the entire tooth, not realizing that most of a tooth, like most of an iceberg, is actually buried from sight. The pulp, on the inside of the tooth, is a soft, blood-filled, sensitive tissue that is immediately enclosed by a hard substance called dentin. The dentin within the root of the tooth is, in turn, enclosed by an outside layer of cementum, a hard, bone-like tissue, while the dentin in the crown is covered by enamel, which is extremely dense. This enamel, on the outside of the crown, is the second-hardest naturally occurring substance; only diamond is harder. Such hardness is of course important in view of the amount of abuse that the teeth take in the chewing of food and the grinding or gnashing of teeth that occurs in many people. It seems paradoxical that such a fabulously hard substance should be such an easy prey to decay.

The pulp inside the crown is housed in a space known as the pulp chamber; that which is in the root area is confined to a narrow passageway called the root canal, that connects with the pulp chamber. The pulp is the remains of the embryological tissue that manufactured the tooth. It has the power to elaborate hard, calcified tissue; it can manufacture and repair tooth structure. (The word *repair* is used here in a special sense; it is not meant to suggest that the pulp can repair and regenerate decayed parts of the tooth.) This function of the pulp is the body's defense against caries, trauma, and irritants. The pulp usually responds to irritation by elaborating new hard tissue, called secondary dentin, on the walls of the root canal and, especially, the pulp chamber. Decay, or a carious lesion, advancing through the crown of a tooth to the pulp chamber, finds this new, hard tissue, secondary dentin, thrown up in its way by the retreating pulp. This race will always be won by the decay, but the defense thrown up by the pulp often gives the dentist enough time to intervene and supply a happy ending to the drama.

5

Dental Pain and Its Control

It is not strange that the popular mind strongly associates dentistry with physical discomfort and even agony. The mouth, where the dentist does his work, is after all a sensitive place, and the teeth and gums can be a source of pain ranging from mild to excruciating, from occasional to chronic. Dental pain can ruin the pleasures of eating, and it can keep one up at night. It can be a twinge or a toothache, a dentist scaling a sensitive tooth or a dentist drilling. But though even the good dentist may be directly responsible for some oral discomfort, it surely is not his fault that so many of his patients come to him only because their mouths hurt them; if they came earlier, or regularly, most of these patients would not have this unpleasant experience, in the dentist's office or out. But as things are, for many people the first association with the word *dentist* is, alas, the notion of pain.

47

Though the pulp is the most common source of dental pain, it is not a nerve. (But when people say "the nerve," they mean the pulp.) A condition of slight irritation of the pulp is called pulpal hyperemia. A hyperemic pulp usually displays sensitivity to cold, and it may be sensitive to the pressure of biting or the action of food juices, especially sugary or acid juices. Hyperemia may be episodic; the symptoms often disappear entirely for long periods of time, returning for briefer episodes. I have had patients whose hyperemia returned twice a year, at the change of seasons, year after year. Most of us have known days when it was impossible to take something cold in the mouth, or to chew ice cream with the front teeth, without experiencing dental pain.

Pulpal inflammation, or pulpitis, produces more acute pain than that which results from pulpal hyperemia. The inflammation may originate in any of several causes: trauma, as from a blow or dental drilling; irritation, because of decay and, possibly, a resulting invasion by bacteria; toxic effects of poorly insulated filling materials; or changes in temperature. Any tissue, including the pulp, tends to swell when it becomes inflamed. But unlike other tissues, which are usually free to expand, the pulp is confined in inflexible walls of dentin. As the inflamed pulp swells, it builds up terrific pressures inside the tooth. It is these pressures which are the direct cause of the most severe dental pain.

The gums may be a source of great pain, particularly if there is infection present. Pain in the gums results from infectious lesions, developing wisdom teeth, and irritations such as denture sores. There are many other causes of mouth pain; the important thing to know is that it is invariably a warning of a real ailment that should be corrected. I have never seen a case of what I could honestly call psychosomatic dental pain. Although on occasion dental pain can be very difficult precisely to locate and correct, such pain is very real and rarely, if ever, psychosomatic in origin.

Mild postoperative pain after any of several different dental procedures is to be expected, and occasionally a patient leaves the dentist's office feeling much worse than when he came in. Postoperative discomfort may prove quite a problem following major restorative work. In case of such pain, and also beforehand, to prevent it, the dentist must devote much thought and energy to the patient's comfort. In periodontal treatment there is usually no pain immediately after a scaling (to remove the calculus, or "tartar," from the visible and the subgingival parts of the teeth), but later in the day there may be discomfort, which rarely lasts more than a day, and can ordinarily be controlled with aspirin. A newly filled tooth, particularly if the filling is deep, is often sensitive to thermal changes, especially to cold, for a few days up to a few weeks. This is because the metal filling, deeply placed, quickly conducts temperature changes deep into the tooth, close to the pulp, causing mild pulpal irritation. The dentist cannot wholly eliminate the possibility of thermal pain, though the likelihood and the severity of any such effect is minimized if he carefully insulates the filling. Again, the discomfort is usually mild enough to be controlled by aspirin. Postoperative pain is sometimes encountered after rootcanal work. Even in this case aspirin will ordinarily keep the discomfort under control. A good rule of thumb is that pain that is too severe to be controlled by aspirin is a sign that something is wrong, and should therefore be brought to the dentist's attention at once, no matter what the time of day or night.

The responsible dentist does not want his patients to suffer; he will wish to alleviate the pain and to consider any implications it may have for the treatment.

There are other possible reasons for postoperative sensitivity of a tooth following restorative procedures. Occasionally the new restoration comes into contact with a previous metal restoration on another tooth. This may lead to the generation of an electric current, a phenomenon called galvanism, which occurs when metals of differing composition are joined by an electrolyte, which in this case is the saliva. A galvanic current may be generated when a silver filling comes close to one of gold, or even to another silver filling whose mercury-silver ratio is not exactly the same. (It is rare that two fillings made at different times have exactly the same metallic proportions.) Such a reaction sometimes induces pain in a newly filled tooth. Over a period of time the symptoms usually disappear; either the tooth accommodates itself to the new situation, or else the two fillings cease to come together in exactly the way which produced the galvanism. If the symptoms prove persistent, they must be brought to the attention of the dentist, who may have to redo the filling, allowing for better insulation.

Traumatic occlusion is an important factor in postoperative sensitivity. If a filling is left too "high," it causes the tooth to come into premature contact with the teeth of the opposite jaw when the patient is chewing. Such malocclusion places great stress on the single high tooth, and it can induce chronic pulpal sensitivity. A tooth that bites too soon must be brought to the attention of the dentist, who will simply grind down the high spot of the filling so as to eliminate the premature biting contact.

Many people unwisely delay a needed visit to the dentist out of fear of being hurt while their teeth are being fixed. This is too bad, both for their oral health and because their fear is largely based on badly out-of-date information, if indeed it is based on anything definite. Undeniably, a dental visit is the occasion for some mild discomfort; it is no joy to sit there with your mouth wide open for so long. On the other hand, the overwhelming majority of dental procedures can today be performed entirely without pain. When anesthesia is in order, the dentist generally prefers to use one of a number of local anesthetics that are available to him. Those used today are derivatives of cocaine, but chemically modified so as to be less toxic and more efficient. Procaine, an early successful cocaine derivative used in dental work, was originally marketed and best known under the famous trademark "Novocaine." Not only are the various local anesthetics currently used in dental work marvelously efficient; they are also remarkably safe.

The local anesthetic is administered by injection. Though the injection itself is sometimes slightly painful, it is rarely very painful, and the benefits to the patient, in his freedom from pain, and to the dentist, in his being able to work on a relaxed and cooperative patient, cannot be overestimated. For a tooth on the upper jaw an injection barely into the tissue by the root of the tooth is usually adequate. This is because the bone of the upper jaw is thin and spongy, so that the anesthetic will soon seep through the bone to the nerve that connects with the root of the tooth. This process is known as infiltration anesthesia. The problem is more difficult for the lower jaw. The roots of the lower teeth are situated in bone that is thicker and denser, and through which the anesthetic will not seep. What is called conduction, or block, anesthesia is needed here. The injection is delivered at the back of the mouth, near the angle of the jaw; it is a deeper injection and is designed to affect the nerve nearer its main source. Such an injection is like turning off a main switch; all of the teeth on the affected side of the lower jaw are anesthetized by the single injection. On the other hand, an infiltration injection on the upper jaw affects only the tooth nearest the site of the injection. The lower-jaw, or mandibular-block, injection also anesthetizes half of the tongue, because the nerve that connects with that part of the tongue lies in the area of the injection.

There are other methods of controlling pain and discomfort. Anxious patients can be given premedication to calm them down. Some dentists work with general anesthesia, rendering the patient completely unconscious before working on him. Still other dentists use what is called "analgesia," which amounts to partial nitrous oxide gas, or "laughing gas," anesthesia. It is generally agreed, however, that local anesthesia administered by injection is the best and most convenient pain suppressant for use in the dental office.

6

Concerning Extractions

It is natural that people should speak in a conversational way to their dentist about their own teeth and about their experiences with other dentists. Many times in my years of practice I have listened sadly as a patient has told me of his lost teeth and the difficulty some other dentist encountered when he took them out. Patients in my dental chair have often made remarks such as these:

"Dentists have always had a hard time pulling my teeth."

"My roots are very long."

"My roots hook around the bone."

"The dentist really sweat over that one."

It seems never to have occurred to these people that, in nearly every case, a tooth with such sturdy roots

53

should never have been extracted. If a tooth was so difficult to remove, if it had such "long" and firmly planted roots, in most instances it would have had sound periodontal support and could have been saved —to give long years of good use.

The person who reaches the age of thirty without having a single tooth extracted is rare indeed, and in this country there were, in the early sixties, according to the National Health Service, twenty million people who had lost all their teeth. More recently it was stated in an article in the *Reader's Digest* (February, 1969) that three out of every ten Americans over thirty-five have no natural teeth left. Against these reports, one of the major themes in this book is that teeth should not be extracted, that ideally people should keep their teeth. Is the reader to conclude that so many Americans can possibly have been victimized by bad dental practice—or are there *often* legitimate reasons for extracting teeth? And may there not be special cases in which an extraction can easily be justified on the ground that the tooth will never be missed, even for esthetic reasons, since it is hidden from view in the back of the mouth?

Let me be blunt: *In general,* teeth should not be extracted, and the great preponderance of extractions are not only unnecessary but wrong. From this it is easy to conclude that most extractions, being unnecessary and wrong, actually constitute malpractice. Extreme though it sounds, this idea is held by many good dentists, and has actually been voiced and published by some. An extraction has a crippling effect on the dentition. Therefore, any extraction that might have been avoided can reasonably be considered malpractice.

The public has long believed that the two major, valid reasons for tooth extraction are infection (abscess) and pain. Yet pain and infection are not clear indications for extraction, and, except in the case of advanced, hopeless periodontal disease, both infection and pain can *always* be successfully treated without extraction. Pulpal infections can be treated with root-canal therapy, and periodontal infections, except the few hopelessly advanced ones, with periodontal therapy. In the allied field of medical practice, the patient's life is never given as the cause of his pain symptom; the physician doesn't treat the pain by burying the patient. In dentistry, similarly, pain is properly treated by removing the cause, be it caries, pulpitis, or whatever, and not by extraction.

Yet there are legitimate reasons for extractions, even when the root is strong. If, therefore, a dentist prescribes an extraction, it does not necessarily follow that he is doing anything improper. In many people the wisdom teeth are the classic exception to the rule that teeth should never (or only rarely) be extracted. For such people the wisdom teeth, or third molars, are vestigial structures for which there is simply not enough room. As the teeth for which there is inadequate space erupt, or come up through the gum, they are seen to be malposed or impacted. Usually pain results; sometimes there is infection; sometimes the next molar is damaged. Since there is not enough room for these teeth, they can never assume a position from which they can contribute functionally to the work of the masticatory apparatus. In short, the wisdom teeth, when malposed or impacted, as they commonly are, contribute nothing but trouble to the mouth. In such cases they are perfect examples of teeth which should be extracted.

Impacted teeth, badly positioned teeth, supernumerary (extra) teeth—these sometimes provide legitimate reasons for extractions even of teeth other than the third molars. And though good orthodontists are not unanimous on this point, it may occasionally be advisable to extract perfectly sound teeth in order to further orthodontic treatment. Most orthodontists now believe that, in some cases, the extraction of certain teeth throughout the dental arch of the young patient is the best method of treating some difficult types of malocclusion. Another special case arises, occasionally, with people who have already had some teeth out, and for whom the dentist is to design a partial denture that has to be anchored to one or more periodontally strong teeth. If the strategic tooth for the anchor, that is, the tooth next to the space to be filled with an artificial tooth or teeth, is too weak to support the denture, that tooth may well have to come out so that a strong tooth beyond it can be used in its place.

People sometimes come to a dentist with teeth in such condition that there is no alternative to extraction. These cases are sometimes the result of the patient's own neglect and sometimes the result of poor dentistry. As a rule, periodontal disease is involved. In the course of such neglected disease, there comes a point beyond which the tooth has become so hopelessly involved, and there is so little bone left around the root, that successful treatment is no longer possible. Though such a condition can usually be headed off by timely care, some patients bring their trouble to the dentist too late for anything better than one or more extractions. More rarely, a tooth that is not periodontally involved is correctly diagnosed as nonrestorable because of extreme decay or fracture. Such cases are extremely rare; a tooth with a periodontally sound root can nearly always be rebuilt almost from nothing. If the root is sound, it can be used as anchorage for a post-crown restoration.

In admittedly difficult cases the so-called strategic value of a tooth is usually taken into account. If a tooth is very necessary to the proper maintenance or restoration of the dentition, the good dentist will go to heroic lengths to save it. On the other hand, he is less inclined to launch into elaborate and very expensive procedures of doubtful prognosis if the tooth has so little strategic importance that the dentition can surely be successfully maintained or restored without it. Extreme, difficult, and expensive treatments of doubtful success may not be justified for less strategic teeth if a satisfactory alternative is available. This should not be misread to mean that a tooth should be readily abandoned merely because it is of only mild strategic importance. Except in the special cases of impacted wisdom teeth, malposed or supernumerary teeth, and so forth, the patient will always, to some degree at least, miss an extracted tooth. For this reason, and for other good reasons, teeth should not be extracted simply on the basis that they will never be missed.

If you are shopping for a dentist, beware of the general practitioner who has built a reputation on the basis of his "painless" extractions. The extraction of a routine tooth is probably the easiest job in dentistry, and it involves the least skill and intelligence. With anesthesia, furthermore, all extractions are supposed to be painless. Remember, the good dentist with a general practice is only rarely called upon to extract a tooth, because he is in the business of saving his patients' teeth, not of squandering them. So steer clear of the neighborhood dentist who is so good at extractions, and go rather to the man who so seldom finds them necessary that most of his patients aren't quite sure whether he pulls them painlessly or not.

Once a tooth has been extracted, the next question is, What should be done now? The answer is, in most cases, replace it promptly. (See chapter on Fixed Bridgework.)

Some people do not understand why a tooth should

be replaced, especially if it be a back tooth whose empty space is not ordinarily seen. But we have said, there is no doubt that the tooth will be missed. Whether or not it is missed on esthetic grounds, its absence will often be felt during mastication. There is a strong chance, also, that the tongue will involuntarily develop a tiresome habit of seeking the empty space. When this happens the patient will be reminded, again and again, of his dental deficiency.

But other considerations are far more important. Teeth, as we have seen, are not absolutely fixed in one position in the jawbone, and may shift position in response to pressures. The dental arch is truly an arch, in the architectural sense, in that each of its many parts gives support directly, or indirectly through other teeth, to each tooth. The teeth are stabilized together in a system such that each tooth depends on each other tooth. Remove just one tooth, and the system comes unhinged. For example, a molar tooth is prevented from drifting forward by the tooth in front of it, and it is prevented from migrating backward by the tooth behind it. But not only do the teeth in one jaw tend to stabilize each other; they also tend to stabilize the facing teeth, in the opposing jaw, into *their* correct positions. The reason an upper molar does not move downward, at least a critical little bit, is that each time the mouth closes, the lower tooth opposing it tends to drive the upper back into position. Other factors, such as the inclinations of the tooth's biting surfaces and the resultant forces generated in biting, and the actions of the cheek, lips, and tongue muscles, all contribute to the equilibrium of the dental arch by preventing the random migration of the teeth.

This equilibrium is destroyed when just one tooth is lost. No longer is the tooth in back of the empty space prevented from moving forward, and so the tooth moves forward. No longer is the tooth in front of it stabilized; therefore it drifts backward. No longer is the tooth above, or below, held in occlusal position, and so this tooth starts to move downward, or upward, into the vacant space. Each movement of each of these teeth will have its own repercussions as the adjoining teeth get into the act and *they* begin to migrate. After a period of time many teeth will, in their turn, join in the migration toward regions of reduced pressure; then we will see the dental arch, which once held all the teeth in proper alignment for best function and best protection against decay and periodontal disease, become irregular in form and inefficient in function. As some teeth begin to tilt, they trap food and become increasingly difficult to clean and keep clean, and the now malformed arch becomes much more susceptible to decay. The forces generated by biting get out of balance, so that great and unaccustomed stresses are transmitted to certain teeth. These pressures will damage the jawbone and the gums and result in periodontal disease.

All this may sound dire, but what follows may prove even worse. The inefficient bite produced by the arch that has been malformed by the loss of a single tooth can alter the biting habits, cause an asymmetry of development of the face and facial muscles, and eventually lead to temporomandibular joint dysfunction with its attendant miseries, including chronic headaches.

One may well ask if all these horrors can possibly result from the extraction of just one molar which isn't even seen from in front, as some laymen would say. The answer is an emphatic Yes! All these things can result and *are very likely to result* from the extraction of just one little molar. But it must be conceded that there are people who have had teeth extracted without having them replaced, and who have suffered relatively little dental or other damage even after several years. Unusually favorable conditions in their mouths provide stability for the remaining teeth and prevent excessive drift. These people are exceptions. For most people, a nonreplaced, extracted tooth will indeed result in the dentally crippling events and symptoms just described.

Some good advice: Except in special cases such as those of impacted wisdom teeth and others already mentioned, do everything possible to keep a tooth that is giving trouble; *the chances are that it is restorable.*

7

The Dental
Examination

Proper dental work cannot be performed without a thorough examination. Besides helping the dentist to form a correct diagnosis and plan of treatment, the examination plays a key role in establishing a tentative fee, so that the patient, instructed by the dentist as to what work is needed, and why, including possible options, can make an informed decision concerning the future of his mouth. A fee should be quoted for this examination beforehand, with the understanding that the fee for the complete dental work cannot be set until after the examination.

There are several components to the complete examination. These include clinical and radiographic examinations, history-taking, study models of the mouth, if desirable, and laboratory tests, if necessary. To attempt to conduct a complete dental examination without X-rays is like trying to watch a movie with the eyes closed; it can't be done. The X-ray examination for an adult usually involves some sixteen to eighteen separate pictures for all of the mouth. X-rays are useful in the identification of conditions such as caries, weakening of bone support (incipient periodontal disease), abscesses, cysts, impacted teeth, retained root tips, subgingival calculus, and bone pathology.

The X-rays are one of the dentist's diagnostic tools, and as such they must remain with him as part of his record of the diagnosis and treatment. The patient pays for the examination, not for the X-rays, which do not belong to him. But any reputable dentist will gladly make them and other records available to any other dentist at the request of the patient.

A great deal has been said about the hazards of radiation. Dental X-rays, properly taken, by licensed personnel using properly designed and inspected equipment, are not hazardous, not even to pregnant women.

The clinical examination is conducted with the eyes, fingers, instruments, and diagnostic aids. With his eyes the dentist checks both the hard tissues (bone and teeth) and the soft tissues (gums, cheeks, tongue, floor of mouth, soft palate). With the fingers the dentist feels the tissues, particularly any irritated areas or lesions; the fingers also check for tooth movement or looseness (mobility). Explorers and probes check for cavities and for depth of periodontal pockets, while the mouth mirror enables the dentist to illuminate and see into concealed areas. Such clinical examination may be started before X-rays are available for study, but should not be completed until they are available for comparison with what can be found clinically in the mouth.

History-taking means interviewing the patient for all information pertinent to the oral and medical condition. It is important for the dentist to know what work has been done in the mouth and to be familiar with the patient's medical history so that he will not use contraindicated procedures. Previous allergic reactions to drugs, and any medical condition such as a cardiac ailment which would require premedication before dental procedures are instituted, are examples of things the dentist must know about before he can safely and intelligently treat his patient. Whether the pulp of a tooth has been treated, or whether orthodontic work has been done, may have a bearing on the work to be done. This is the type of information that the dentist should get from his history-taking. Patients with certain types of problems may require additional diagnostic procedures. Thus, it may be useful to have study impressions taken for patients with occlusal disharmony, or bad bite. The study models of the teeth made from these impressions may be of great assistance in correcting the bite or in planning a restoration. Laboratory tests are made when the dentist suspects a systemic factor, possibly disease or metabolic imbalance, bearing on the oral condition.

In common with all phases of good dentistry, a proper dental examination takes time; it simply cannot be completed in a few minutes. The quickie examination is a specialty of Dr. Poorwork, who rarely takes the time to do anything right.

A good part of the dentist's responsibility at the time of the examination is to tell the patient, in clear terms, what his oral condition is, and to explain carefully what can and should be done, why it should be done, and what might be expected if it were not done. This education of the patient does not stop here, but continues to be the never-ending responsibility of the dentist. After reporting to the patient, the dentist may suggest alternative treatments and fees. Sometimes the most desirable treatment is beyond the patient's means, and a less desirable, but still satisfactory treatment is agreed upon. Of course, it is up to the reputable dentist to see that whatever treatment is adopted is sound, and that no unsound procedures are used.

Is such a complete examination necessary every time the patient comes back for a check-up? Of course not. Recall check-ups, once there has been a thorough initial examination, need not be so extensive. For example, X-rays that show the tips of the roots are not routinely necessary; the conditions they reveal do not develop in six months. For some patients the dentist does not take any X-rays more frequently than every one or two years, while for others it may be advisable to check for decay by means of X-rays every six months. But every several years, at the discretion of the dentist, a complete examination should be given again.

8

The Drill, Some Gimmicks, and Factory - Style Dentistry

Many people tend to judge a dentist by the array of machinery in his shop rather than by his professional results. Some select their dentist because he has what they call "the painless drill," some because he has "sweet air," some because he has stereo, and even some because he has four nurses. "I go to Dr. P," one person says, "He has all the latest equipment."

The technological revolution of the past two decades has inevitably involved dentistry, which depends so much upon machinery to achieve its results. In these years a multitude of new approaches and styles in dental equipment have become available. While most of the new devices are simply variations of old ones, some represent significant advances in ease of operation for the dentist and increased comfort for the patient. The dentist is therefore well advised to install dental equipment that incorporates these legitimate advances. But, for the patient, shiny dental equipment provides no assurance that his dentist performs the best or the most modern dentistry. In fact, much of the old-fashioned, inadequate, and downright bad dentistry performed today is done with brand-new equipment, and the so-called painless or high-speed drill is one of the most abused dental instruments ever used. Given enough time and effort, on the other hand, *all* of the results of good, modern dentistry can be obtained with old fashioned equipment.

The Drill

If there is a phrase which, more than any other, evokes the traditional horror and fear of the dentist, that phrase is "the drill." Invested with emotional dynamite though it may be, the drill is the most valuable instrument in the dentist's armamentarium. Without it, the modern dentist is virtually helpless and could not properly accomplish any of the basic restorative procedures. During the past fifteen years this vital instrument has been the focus of the most important technological changes in dentistry.

The dentist's drill is much like any drill. It consists of a machine that operates a rotary drill bit, which may be a bur, disk, or stone. These bits are employed in the removal of decay and undermined tooth structure, and in extending, grooving, bevelling, and shaping teeth to receive restorations and to adjust occlusion. The drill also plays an important role in endodontic, periodontic, orthodontic, and surgical procedures. Should a dentist's drill need repairs, he may as well close up shop until they are done.

For half a century no major improvements were made in this drill, which operated at speeds of roughly ten to ten thousand revolutions per minute. Then, in the

1950's, an ultra-high-speed drill was introduced with speeds upwards of 100,000 rpm. Today there are drills which operate at speeds upwards of 300,000 rpm. The new drills have eased the dentist's burden significantly, but there is an enormous misunderstanding in the public mind as to just what the drills can and cannot do.

First a brief word on the technology of these instruments. The old, conventional drill was belt-driven, usually by an electric motor, though old-timers and front-line Army dentists will remember a foot-pedal-powered drill. Among the new drills some of the earlier ones were belt-driven by an intricate system of tiny belts and pulleys which stepped up the speed from the source of power into the high-speed range. Subsequent drills are driven by air in a turbine arrangement; some use an ingenious air-bearing system. The use of transistorized control boxes has brought remarkable results in miniaturization and efficiency.

The conventional slow-speed drill used burs of steel and stones and disks of Carborundum, sandpaper, and other abrasives. These materials are inadequate at high speeds. The new burs are of extra-hard tungsten carbide steel; stones are made of diamond chips. At high speeds the stones and burs do not cut so much as they shear and chip. The feel of the drill in the hands of the dentist is different. To him, it is as if he were gently wiping off areas of the tooth, rather than forcibly cutting and grinding it. The drilling process seems much smoother to the patient, and he is less likely to feel that the dentist is leaning on his tooth.

At these high speeds the heat of friction becomes a problem. Heat may damage the pulp of the tooth, perhaps even to the extent that the pulp will be destroyed and root canal work made necessary. As a precaution against excessive heat, all the high-speed drills employ a water spray which plays on the tooth while the drill is in operation. Even with this precaution, the dentist must be careful to touch the tooth only intermittently with the drill and to avoid sustained pressure on any tooth.

Many dentists, the author included, feel that no drill operated at high speeds is suitable for the removal of deep decay. Removal of deep decay is partly a matter of "feel" in the hands of the dentist. Often there is no room for error, since there is only an extremely thin layer of sound tooth structure between the decay and the pulp. It is important to preserve this layer; the tooth has less of a chance of uneventful recovery without it. Should this thin shield be perforated, then work on the tooth will have to be complicated by an endodontic procedure. This may be a pulp-capping or a more complicated procedure. Great pains must therefore be taken to avoid involvement of the pulp. In recognition of this, dental supply manufacturers are now including various low-speed devices with their high-speed set-ups.

Certain types of work can be speeded up considerably with a high-speed drill, particularly work involving bulk reduction of tooth structure. Removal of metal fillings and inlays, once a tiresome, bone-jarring job, is easy with the new instruments. The preparation of the teeth for major restorations, such as crowns, jackets, and inlays has become much easier for the dentist, and it is easier on the patient, too. With this equipment, the patient is relatively free from the old oppressive, rattling sensation, but though it is often called the painless drill, it is usually anything but painless. Even with this instrument, deep drilling without anesthesia for the preparation of a restoration is very painful to the average person. However, shallow drilling can often be done painlessly, and badly decayed teeth may be partially excavated without pain. Now, perhaps, one can see why the high-speed drill is right up Dr. Poorwork's alley. He uses his brand-new "painless" drill to make a perfunctory pass at the tooth, excavating some decay painlessly in a very short time, and then he fills the tooth. In this manner Dr. Poorwork can complete the entire operation in just a few minutes, painlessly and without anesthesia. Thus he saves himself time and enhances his reputation as a painless dentist and a man who "has the latest." Such improper use of high-speed equipment by Poorworks is very widespread.

Two other modern dental devices can be mentioned here, though they are not drills. One is the Airdent. This operated much on the principle of a sandblaster, a slurry of metallic powder being sprayed against the tooth to effect cutting and grinding. It did not work too well, and never attained widespread use. The other device is the Cavitron. This works electrically, developing vibrations of supersonic frequencies. The machine was not successful as a cutting instrument, but it has been modified and is now used by many dentists for cleaning tooth surfaces, as an aid in periodontal scaling, and for the condensation of silver amalgam fillings. Unlike the Airdent, the Cavitron has legitimate dental uses. But though it will not do a complete and effective periodontal scaling, some dentists do use it for that purpose.

Some Gimmicks

The word *gimmick* suggests a type of concealed method or subtle trick that is used to sell something that the customer may not need. The universal lure of gain has fostered gimmicks everywhere. In dentistry there are gimmicks in equipment, as we have seen, and in operative procedures, medications, office furnishings, public relations, practice management, and even in fees. And these gimmicks are indeed effective.

Anesthesia is a major field for dental gimmickry. Any dentist desiring to promote his practice is eager to let the word get around that he never hurts anybody. "Painless" dentistry can be accomplished by inadequate cavity preparation or by the use of anesthesia. "Sweet-air" is a child-directed euphemism for nitrous oxide gas, an anesthetic gas. Nitrous oxide gas is often used to induce partial rather than complete general anesthesia. This effect, called analgesia, has been described as a condition in which the pain of drilling is still present but the patient, who is only semiconscious, doesn't much care. Analgesia can be used to prepare the way for an injection of a local anesthetic, or it can be used instead of local anesthesia. I confess I am prejudiced against this latter use. In work with children, the need to attend constantly to the gas inhalator only complicates the difficult task of filling the child's tooth. With adults, the method is less effective in reducing pain than it is with children. Furthermore, all examples of dental work I have seen which I knew to have been done with analgesia have been poor dentistry; the technique seems to be a favorite with many Poorworks. These observations explain my prejudice against analgesia. I use the word *prejudice* advisedly. Many reputable dentists use analgesia, and theoretically there is no reason why high-quality work cannot be done using the technique. But if such work has been done with analgesia, I haven't seen it.

Audio analgesia had somewhat of a vogue among the gimmick dentists some years ago. The hypothesis of audio analgesia was that if all outside noise were excluded from the patient's hearing, and if he was subjected through earphones to what was called "white noise," a state not unlike hypnosis would be produced in which dental procedures, including extractions, could be carried out painlessly. White noise sounds somewhat like escaping steam or the loud hiss of interstation static on a powerful radio. Taking the white-noise theory as fact, manufacturers assembled and hastily marketed elaborate hi-fi systems which promised to deliver to the patients, via earphones, muzak-type stereo music in times of little stress, and pure white noise, as needed, for pain. Audio analgesia was a pleasant enough idea which simply didn't work, except, reportedly, in the case of a few individuals who must have been very suggestible. After the collapse of the white-noise fad, many dentists kept the apparatus for its music, in the belief that their patients would rather hear music than the noise of drilling. But this too had its drawback: Some found that treatment became less efficient because the music prevented the patient from hearing the dentist tell him to open wider or rinse out.

Medications can be made into gimmicks; this is more common in the practice of medicine, but it is also seen in dentistry. Some patients with a sore or a minor discomfort may be disappointed if the doctor doesn't "put something on it." This "something" may be entirely worthless in treating the condition, but as long as it tastes or smells like medicine, the patient may be satisfied. The canker sore, or apthous ulcer, provides a good example in dentistry. The apthous ulcer can be annoying and even painful and, much like the common cold, runs its course in seven to ten days. No satisfactory treatment has yet been devised for it. To keep the patient happy, the dentist may apply some medicine to make it better, and perhaps to justify a fee. In such cases a topical anesthetic is usually the medication used; this numbs the sore for a few minutes, after which the dentist can hope that the patient will forget about his trouble, at least for a little while longer. But, of course, the medication will not contribute to the healing of the sore. Gentian violet is another medication often used as a gimmick. This is a strong purple dye that probably has no medical properties whatever, despite its widespread use. Its major value is its deep color. The patient, seeing his gums turn purple with the "medication," is led to believe that something is really being done for him, and indeed it is: His attention is being diverted from his complaint to his gruesomely stained gums.

The dentist's public relations is laden with gimmickry. The Code of Ethics prohibits advertising; it also prohibits any public statements on dentistry which have not been approved by the society. Public criticism of any dentist or of any dental practices is particularly forbidden. With these restrictions, a dentist seeking to promote his practice must be very careful. If a patient asks why his dentist takes five times as long and charges twice as much as Dr. Poorwork across the street, the dentist must not even hint that Dr. Poorwork cannot be doing proper dentistry. Instead, he may only try to convince his patient that his own work is very good. If the patient concludes that the dentist is an inefficient bumbler who charges outrageous prices, that is just too bad for the dentist. Of course, the dentist can say that his work is the very best, but again he finds himself in the weak position of not being able to characterize Dr. Poorwork's five-minute dentistry as being even slightly inferior. Deprived of the right to say, "My work is superior to the work of many other dentists, because, unlike them, I give each task the time needed to do it correctly," he may turn to gimmicks, which will be less pertinent, but may nonetheless serve to impress the patient.

Diplomas and other documents are one form of such gimmickry. Nearly every dentist displays his dental diploma and license, and some dental offices have walls covered with diplomas, citations, and so on, designed to impress the patient with the dentist's massive qualifications. I have seen the damndest things in these displays, all beautifully laminated in plastic and framed: High-school diplomas, Army discharges, fraternity citations, and even a commendation won by the doctor's wolfhound at the dog show. An extension of this sort of nonsense is the trick of the dentist with a general practice who somehow lets the word get out that he is a specialist, or that his work is special in some way. These men often have an imposing office and the imperious bearing to go with the fatuous citations on the wall. Of course, such dentists are not specialists, a specialist being a man who specifically limits his practice to a single phase of dentistry.

Dentists, who are not permitted to advertise, have nevertheless found many "ethical" ways of getting their names before the public. For example, there are the opening-of-practice announcements which the new dentist may send to friends, acquaintances, colleagues, and others. There are also the announcements of the formation of associations and the announcements of going into a legitimate specialty. Dentists are permitted to send periodic recall reminders or appointment notices to their own patients only. They are also permitted to send greeting cards to patients and friends. Though these are about the only legitimate ways a dentist has to keep his name before the public, still other, more questionable methods are used. Some dentists give out medals for "bravery" to young patients. Predictably, the dentist's name is prominently engraved on each medal. Dentists give children pencils on which the following inspiring message is printed: "I have been to Dr. Poorwork." Toys, rings, even lollipops (!) are also handed to child patients. Adults are given pamphlets on oral hygiene, and toothbrushes with the dentist's name on them. Pamphlets entitled "The Care of Your

Denture" have Dr. Poorwork's name on the cover, and denture-cleaning brushes have his name stamped in gold.

Few patients have any notion of the real basis of the dental fee, and it is for this reason that fees often involve deception. Patients may be led to believe that they are charged per filling, so much for X-rays, so much for a cleaning, and so on. But what constitutes a filling or a cleaning? Are five X-rays half the price of ten X-rays? Does a filling which takes an hour "cost" as much as a filling that takes fifteen minutes? What does a dentist mean when he says that there are three fillings in one tooth? Although commonly held notions about fees are absurd, most dentists do not disturb these false ideas, for fear that the patient may worry about the size of his bill. In order to establish even a realistic fee, therefore, the dentist feels compelled to resort to gimmickry, and he is careful not to tell the patient the true basis of the fee.

The hottest thing in dentistry these days is a gimmicky field called practice management. This is the pious term given to the efforts of the dentist to make money by building up his practice. Of course, there is nothing wrong with the principle that dentists must make money. The inexperienced practitioner does need some instruction in how to keep his office running smoothly and how to deal with his patients so that they not only pay what they owe him, but they come back to him. Dentists, like other people, have to make a living; if they did not, there would be no dentists. The problem is one of perspective. Judging by the shop-talk of many dentists, one would think that practice management, not teeth or oral health, was the chief interest of dentistry.

There was a time when serious scientific articles and

discussions of dental problems monopolized the reading time of professional men, but it seems that today much professional reading is in the field of practice management. There are a number of handbooks on the subject, and several years ago there appeared a dental journal devoted wholly to it. The magazine caught on, and before long other such publications were launched. More recently *Oral Hygiene,* one of the oldest established dental journals, changed its editorial policy and even its name (to *Dental Economics*) in order to devote itself entirely to practice management. What do we find in these magazines? Most of the articles are on methods and tricks to enlarge the practice and make more money from it. There are articles on how to get patients, how to keep them, how to present and sell suggested treatments, how to utilize nurses, technicians, and secretaries to the best advantage, how to lay out an office, how to "upgrade" the practice (English translation: how to raise fees), how to work more efficiently, how to bill, how to make collections, and so forth.

I have before me the January, 1969, issue of *Dental Management,* a typical practice-management magazine. It is large in format, slickly produced, and runs to 112 pages, which are mostly advertising. The eight articles listed in the "Table of Contents," together with most of the short, teasing quotations that accompany the listings, are as follows:

Your Tax Consultant—"Every doctor needs one. Here's how to find the man that's right for you."

Solutions to Your Toughest Collection Problems —"There's no security on the credit you advance to patients. Everything depends on their willingness and ability to pay . . . and your ability to size it up."

The Games Patients Play—"More than dentistry

goes on in the treatment room. Here's a scorecard to help you recognize the players."

Variable Annuity: Flexible Dollars for Your Retirement. . . .

Tax Questions and Answers.

'So That's How They Hooked Dr. X!'—"By using something called the 'net worth' method. It's the Treasury's sharpest weapon, but few doctors know how it can be turned against them."

Switch to Double-Entry Books?—"Maybe you should if your practice warrants it. This article will help you decide."

Opportunities in Commodity Trading—"Ninety per cent of those who start in this field drop out within two years. First you learn how to lose money gracefully; then you learn how to make it."

In addition, the magazine contains features with information on stocks, retirement funds, taxes and tax deductions, insurance, and so on. Aside from such pieces and all the advertising, there is nothing else in this issue of a representative practice-management magazine. Its editorial columns do not contain any serious material on the treatment of dental disease, on fixing teeth, or on dental research.

Of the eight articles, only "The Games Patients Play" has anything at all to do with patients in treatment. The author of the piece, Donald F. Rohlfs, tries to analyze the "transactions" between dentist and patient by using the method of Dr. Eric Berne's popular book, *Games People Play*. The content and flavor of the article are sufficiently illustrated by this extract:

It might go like this: Mom comes in with one of her difficult ones, and you knock yourself out controlling the brat and finally accomplish something. Mom is amazed that you got anything done at all. In fact, she is so pleased that she makes you this offer: "You know, Doc, I've got a large family and if you give us a break, I'll send 'em all to you, you lucky dog."

This is her calculating Adult speaking, Doc, and if you don't want to be a loser you'd better get your Adult into the game right now! Because here's what your Parent might think: Poor thing, she's got an awful lot to put up with. That kid really needed direction and help, so his brothers and sisters must too. After all, I'm here to help."

The article goes flippantly on to make clear why you must not allow, God forbid, the intrusion of a humane thought to turn you aside from the main goal of dentistry according to the Gospel of Practice Management. In a word, the sacred goal you must always keep in view is, obviously, money. Mustn't begin to feel kindly toward a mother with seven kids "if you don't want to be a loser," Doc!

I have read articles, examined brochures, and heard lectures on practice management whose strident tones would have made Babbitt recoil. Huckstering phrases abound: "Personal power—the golden thread of effective dental practice!" "I reached the magic one-hundred-thousand figure, thanks to you!" (Yes, this means $100,000 yearly from a dental practice.) "This is the year! Prepare yourself for the great leap forward! Here's how!" It may be hard to believe that such nonsense is typical of practice management but, alas, it is. There are dentists who are always professing concern about the "public image" of dentistry. They would do well to take a critical look at practice management. Not long ago a layman asked me whether it was dentistry's purpose to care for people's health or to make money. I told him the purpose was to care for people's dental health. I hope he never gets to read one of the practice-management magazines.

Factory-Style Dentistry

An important movement among dentists aims to make dentistry more efficient, to make it possible to perform dental work more quickly and still, ostensibly, maintain the highest standards of quality.[1] To this end, new concepts of practice have been introduced which, in some cases, have led to what has been called factory-style dentistry. A caricature of a factory practice might include several operating rooms, several chairs, several secretaries and assistants, a dental hygienist, and perhaps several dentists—or one *very* fast-moving dentist who flits from patient to patient. The office layout is the result of "scientific" studies which have eliminated as much waste time and motion as possible. Record-keeping and billing employ the latest automated techniques. In rapid succession, the patient may have X-rays taken by one girl, a "cleaning" done by another, and an injection from a dentist, who quickly disappears to work on another patient until the anesthesia takes. The whole scene is one of fantastic efficiency of motion: Patients streaming in and out, nurses interviewing, ushering, collecting money, and sharp-eyed dentists dashing about from room to room. But all this activity should not dazzle or overimpress the patient. For him, the only important consideration is whether he will receive proper care.

---

[1] I consider that there are only two qualities of dentistry: The highest standard, and inadequate.

Factory-style dentistry is hailed by some as the wave of the future, and it must not be summarily dismissed. Scientific studies of the quality of care provided by private factory-style practices are not available, partly because the concept of streamlined dentistry is still young, but it is not too soon to make some critical comments. It has been my personal observation that factory practices lead to bad work. Because of my observations, I am inclined to believe that superefficient, factory dentistry will never lead to the best dental care. But, as we shall see in this chapter and elsewhere, it is important that we look further into this subject.

No doubt there is a great deal of "wasted" time in the typical one-man practice. Were this wasted time put to productive use, the dentist could treat more patients and make more money. A word of caution is in order here: The practice-management manuals use the term *productive* to mean productive of fees, and they use *wasted* to suggest a lost chance to make money. But *productive* can also mean productive of good dental work, and *wasted* can mean a lost opportunity to perform work for a patient. In either case, wasted time does exist for every dentist, and the "efficient" style of practice aims to eliminate it. But is wasted time really wasted? The time that might be wasted waiting for an injection to take can be used to discuss the treatment with the patient, to answer his questions, to check on oral hygiene, to organize dental instruments needed in the procedure, to study the situation prior to the procedure, to arrange appointment schedules, or merely to chat for a moment with the patient to establish better rapport with him.

An efficient dental practice can indeed eliminate much supposedly wasted time, and perhaps speed up some procedures, and still maintain high standards, but always to run at peak efficiency is too much strain for a man required to make important decisions for other human beings all day, every day. For flesh-and-blood dentists, a little leeway for waste and inefficiency is necessary! Otherwise, decision-making becomes machine-like and the quality of care suffers from a lack of human consideration. If streamlined practice can complete the average two-surface filling in fifteen minutes (no wasted time!), and the schedule allows fifteen minutes for the procedure, what happens when unexpected difficulties arise, and the filling takes a half hour or more? Will the dentist, faced with the pressure of his scheduling, throw the schedule severely out of line by spending the necessary extra time with the patient, or will he settle for a job which is "good enough," i.e. inadequate, in order to finish in the allotted time? In my own practice I find that some leeway in estimated time for each appointment is indispensable. Merely having the extra time available, even when the patient does not need it, takes a good deal of the pressure off me and contributes to my ability to do my best work.

So far we have been discussing the ultraefficient practices which make an effort to do good work. But I have observed that most factory-style, multi-chair offices have been set up not to produce good work, but to perform Poorwork-style dentistry at a high rate of speed. In some cities these offices have been set up in slum areas to exploit the relatively generous Medicaid fee scales and the great availability of Medicaid patients. (Medicaid fee scales are generous only by Poorwork standards. For their hasty and sloppy work, the Poorworks usually charge less than good dentists can afford to charge for their good work.)

Despite all these considerations, the multiple-chair type of practice undoubtedly is the wave of the future. If rationally and humanely engineered, it is theoretically the best way to practice dentistry. The catch lies in the words "if rationally and humanely engineered." A practice set up solely to increase production, to run at top efficiency, and to make barrels of money, loses sight of what ought to be the first objective of *all* practice —to take the best care of the patients by performing the best possible dental service. And despite my own negative observations, mentioned above, even I believe that the multiple-chair concept does indeed offer the best framework for the future practice of dentistry, and for many reasons, which are elaborated in the chapter "New Directions." But it cannot be said too often that the ultimate criterion for judging the success of a dental practice—indeed, the sole criterion, if only one is to be used—must be the dental health of the patients. "Is the dental work successful? Do the patients keep their teeth?" These are the critical questions that we must ask when evaluating a dental practice.

9

Dental Decay and Its Major Treatment: The Filling

It is impossible to write at length about dentistry without referring repeatedly to decay, or caries. Tooth decay is the most prevalent disease of all mankind; only a minute fraction of the world's people are free of it; it is even more common than the common cold. With caries being so universally distrubuted, with such limitless opportunity to study it, one might imagine that by now medical science would have learned all about this major scourge. Alas, the innermost secrets of caries, like those of the cold, have so far eluded all our investigations.

The Causes and Prevention of Decay

The cause of caries has been the subject of the most intensive speculation and research. Present theory involves acids, dental plaque, bacteria, food residue,

82

salivary pH, and bad oral hygiene; this last, of course, relates to all the other factors, each of which has been implicated and is known to be present during the formation of carious lesions. But the exact role, if any, of each agent and of possible others remains a mystery. Briefly and simply, the current thinking on the causes of decay is as follows: The tooth is constructed of both organic and inorganic elements. The organic (tissue) elements serve as a matrix about which form the hard, calcified, inorganic elements. In caries, the inorganic tooth structure is dissolved by acids, while the organic structure is destroyed by the action of proteolytic enzymes. The acids implicated in the decalcification of the hard tooth structure are probably metabolic by-products of bacteria feeding on food residues, first, and on organic tooth structure, later. The dental plaque, a complex composite of debris on the surface of a poorly-cleaned tooth, probably plays a prominent role; it harbors colonies of microorganisms in intimate contiguity with the tooth.

Little as we know about the exact causes of caries, we do know quite a bit concerning its progress and prevention. We know, for example, that caries progresses at different rates in different environments. Some individuals, for a variety of reasons, experience rapid rates of tooth decay, while in other mouths decay proceeds very slowly. In some individuals a very small cavity will not change for years, while in others an identical lesion may reach serious proportions in a matter of months. There is no doubt that the mouth chemistry and composition of the saliva play an important role in these differences. It is most likely, for instance, that decay will proceed apace in an acid medium. Every dental student has seen a demonstration of a jar of soda-pop in which a recently extracted, carious tooth is placed; within a few days the tooth almost dissolves away.

(Think of this the next time your caries-prone child has a soda!) If one's saliva tends to be on the acid side, decay will probably occur more rapidly. People whose saliva tends to be less acid are more resistant to decay, but are more prone to calculus formation and resultant periodontal disease. These statements about saliva and decay are over-simplifications subject to many scientific reservations, but they do nevertheless convey some idea of the relation of oral chemistry to tooth pathology.

An individual may be caries-prone for many reasons. His saliva may be chemically conducive to caries formation. His oral hygiene may be slovenly, permitting food debris to accumulate. This food debris begins to decompose in the mouth, both from the action of mouth bacteria and from salivary digestive enzymes. The decomposing food particles form a ready medium for colonies of acid-forming bacteria and contribute to the building of the dental plaque, considered by many authorities a prime cause of caries and major irritant causing periodontal damage. In fact, poor oral hygiene with all its ramifications is undoubtedly the most important cause of dental caries.

Some people's saliva may have physical as well as chemical characteristics conducive to caries. A viscous, mucilaginous saliva retains food in the mouth and aids in forming tacky materia alba (whitish, slimy food residues) which adheres to the necks of teeth and the gingival margin of the tissues. On the other hand, a serous, watery saliva tends to wash away food debris and thus to lower the incidence of caries. Diet can be another important factor. It is well known that there are statistically significant relationships between the severity of caries in certain populations and the diets of these populations. The rich diets of modern western man, high in refined sugars and carbohydrates, are conducive to caries. Refined carbohydrates—sugars, starches, and flours—are exactly the types of food which readily form the tacky food residues that are hard to remove and that, with bacterial and enzymatic help, quickly produce acid by-products which attack the teeth. But thorough and *prompt* oral hygiene procedures after eating theoretically reduce if not eliminate the caries-producing activity of the modern diet. It is the presence of these foodstuffs *in the mouth,* not in the stomach, that is dangerous.

There has been some talk concerning the usefulness of foods which tend to keep a mouth clean; sometimes these are called "detergent foods." We know that refined carbohydrates tend to form food debris and materia alba. Detergent foods such as crunchy vegetables, crisp salads, and so on do not form materia alba, and they actually scour away some food debris. But such talk is rendered academic when the principles of sound oral hygiene are applied.

It may come as a surprise to most people that, from the nutritional standpoint, diet is *not* a factor in dental caries. The ingestion of fresh fruit and milk does *not* reduce the incidence of caries; in the absence of good oral hygiene, in fact, they too can contribute to the decaying process. Though adequate nutrition is essential to the continued health of every child and every adult, nutrition has nothing to do with dental decay. Again, it is the food remaining in the mouth which decays teeth, not the food in the stomach. Nutrition can play a part in other mouth disorders and in periodontal disease, but not in caries. Even severe childhood nutritional deficiencies rarely affect the teeth. A calcium deficiency in childhood, for example, results in rickets, a weakening of the bones, but rarely affects the calcification of the teeth. Ignorance about oral hygiene and lack of knowledge concerning proper dental treatment are to blame for poor or lost teeth, not early poverty and parents who failed to provide a proper diet. It is true that some high-fever diseases of early childhood may interfere with the calcification of developing teeth. Yet this condition, rare enough in the United States today, is hardly ever a factor in dental caries even when it exists.

Although most adult Americans do not practice really good oral hygiene, with knowledge and effort these adults can easily correct their habits. The problem is more serious with children, who do not have sufficient manual dexterity or self discipline to maintain good oral hygiene. Many children show patterns of "continuous eating"; they are always chewing on something, be it fruit, bread, or lollypops. Since continuous brushing is not feasible, parents should strive to break a child's continuous-eating pattern, because it is particularly insidious in causing serious caries. Because of their poor oral hygiene, control of diet in young children is especially important. They should not be given highly cariogenic foods. Candies, particularly hard, sucking candies, should be guarded against, since they produce a sugary acid component in the saliva for long periods of time. I cringe whenever I see a child with a lollypop, and yet I know of dentists who give lollypops to children as a reward for being good! There is nothing worse than a lollypop for a caries-prone child. Sugar-laden chewing gum and soda pop are other prime offenders. Remember how fast a carious tooth will dissolve in a test tube of soda? The tooth does not rot as fast in the mouth, of course, because of the acid-neutralizing capabilities of the saliva, but if the destruction is slower, it is just as sure.

Observers of differing ethnic groups in different parts of the world have noticed that the incidence of caries can vary sharply among different populations, and

have always concluded that differences in diet accounted for such variations. This is undoubtedly true; but
in the presence of uniform, proper oral hygiene habits
among these populations the effect of the dietary differences on the incidence of caries would be minimized.
The English are reputed to have more than their share
of bad teeth. Undoubtedly their sugar-laden diet, ac-
cented with refined pastries and breads, contributes
heavily to the caries problem, but more important still
are the considerations of poor oral hygiene and poor
dental care. My few opportunities to observe English
dental work have led me to conclude that preventive
and restorative dentistry are at a low level in England.

The role of heredity in dental disease is imperfectly
understood. Although the son may seemingly "inherit"
his father's buck teeth, bad gums, or high rate of decay,
it is more likely that learned habits of muscular patterns, facial mannerisms, diet, and oral hygiene are
more important factors than genetics. Of course the
family's neglect of dental care, or the quality of the
dental care sought are important; neglect and Dr.
Poorwork are the biggest causes of bad teeth.

Though experience indicates that the teeth of some
people are constitutionally more disposed to the ravages of decay than the teeth of more fortunate others, it
seems more accurate to say that some *mouths* are more
prone to decay than others, and for many reasons
(chemistry, saliva, oral hygiene, and so on). There is
no longer any doubt that teeth with more fluoride in
their composition are considerably more resistant to
decay than those with less fluoride. But there is no such
thing as "soft teeth"; all teeth are *very* hard. In fact,
tooth enamel is the second hardest naturally occurring
substance known to nature, second only to diamonds
in hardness, and much harder than such materials as
iron, gold, and porcelain. The expression *soft teeth* is

often used erroneously to refer to teeth in mouths demonstrating a high proclivity to caries, usually because
of factors such as mouth chemistry or poor oral hygiene, but *never* because of the softness of the teeth.
This term is often taken literally by the patient who
despairs of ever being able to keep his teeth and who
resigns himself to early dentures. "Soft teeth" is a favorite expression of Dr. Poorwork to explain why his
work so often "goes bad." Of course, *his* patients have
every reason to despair about the future of their teeth,
but not because they are soft.

Another old-wives' tale that needs refutation concerns the relationship between the calcium requirements of the embryo and the oral health of the pregnant
woman. "The baby took all the calcium out of my teeth,
and so I lost them." I have heard this too often, and it
is never true. The developing embryo does not take
calcium from the mother's teeth to satisfy its requirements. If the mother's diet is deficient in calcium, the
calcium requirements of the embryo will be met first,
and the mother may lose some calcium from her *bones,*
but not from her teeth. That mothers should blame
their infants for their tooth troubles probably has emotional origins. Some pregnant women, particularly
those in their first pregnancy, are so concerned with
their swelling belly and the contents thereof that they
tend to let themselves go, and neglect their oral hygiene. Of course, cavities result. In other cases it may
simply be coincidence; the age at which a woman is
likely to be pregnant may coincide with the age range
at which people who have neglected their teeth and do
not receive proper care begin to have them extracted.
It is also possible that the mother's resentment toward
the infant who has brought such inconvenience to her
life plays a part in the false accusation that the child
"ruined" her teeth. In any case, this complaint is never

heard from mothers who have practiced good oral hygiene and received competent dental care before, during, and after pregnancy.

The Treatment of Dental Decay

The treatment of dental caries can be generally summed up in the rule: Remove caries completely and restore the teeth to form and function. Of course, this is easier said than done. Removal of the decay, difficult and delicate job that it can be, is the simpler task. The restorative considerations and work can be exceedingly complex. Usually a tooth can be salvaged if nothing more than a sound root stump remains, but there are few times when so little is left of the root that extraction is the only solution. In these few cases the restorative problem involves replacing the missing tooth. If the tooth is restorable, but the caries involves the pulp, then rootcanal work is required. If the crown of the tooth is badly broken down by the caries, then a full crown or large cast restoration is needed. Finally, if the caries has not done such major damage, we remain in the realm of the most common of dental restorations, the filling. (Let us be clear that a cavity is a carious lesion, a defect, a hole in a tooth, something that must be corrected, while the filling is the restoration, the treatment, the correction of the defect. Strange as it may seem, these two terms often get confused.)

The steps in the preparation and construction of a silver amalgam filling are outlined in chapter one. Essentially: (1) Decay must be completely removed, and the tooth prepared to receive the filling by removing all weakened tooth structure; (2) a soundly engineered pattern must be cut in the tooth to hold the filling strongly and to minimize the possibility of future decay at that tooth surface; and (3) the filling is then carefully placed in the tooth. These procedures take time, but if carefully carried through they can be very successful. A properly made filling may last indefinitely, while a badly made filling almost invariably fails.

Many materials have been used to make fillings. These include various metals, cements, compositions, and plastics, but as yet dentistry does not have a completely satisfactory restorative material. To be absolutely perfect, a filling material must have many important qualities:

1. It should be esthetic. It should look exactly like part of the tooth which was replaced, both in form and color.
2. It must be non-poisonous.
3. It must be such that it can be readily manipulated in the mouth. High-fusing porcelain looks good and would make an excellent material for some types of fillings, but since it must be baked at temperatures well over one thousand degrees Fahrenheit it cannot be used for fillings that are to be shaped in the mouth.
4. It must be resistant to abrasion, both from the wear of chewing and at contact points.
5. The material must be stable. A filling must not react chemically with anything likely to enter the mouth. It must not break down with temperature changes or the passage of time.
6. It must have good crushing and edge strength. The forces of mastication are tremendous. A filling must be resistant to breaking, crushing, and chipping.
7. The material should not flow. The filling, once placed, should not flow over the edges when subjected to stress.

8. The ideal material would not conduct temperature changes or electrical impulses. Thermal and electrical shock can be damaging to the pulp of a tooth.

9. The material must have a favorable coefficient of expansion. The coefficient of expansion is a measurement of the amount a material will expand when heated. If the filling material expands more or less than the tooth structure, then with each change of temperature in the mouth, when hot coffee or a cold drink is taken, the filling and the tooth will change dimensions at different rates. This will result in filling margins that leak, and may lead to the actual popping out of the filling.

10. The material must be insoluble in the oral fluids.

One can see that the selection of a material with which to fill teeth is no simple matter. What may be the best material we have thus far is not esthetic and is not easily worked; this is gold foil. A gold foil filling is very difficult to place, but once properly installed it is virtually indestructable. Gold foil is little used today because of the difficulty and expense involved and because of the esthetic objections to gold in front of the mouth.

Silver amalgam is probably the most commonly used filling material today, and, properly used, a very good material it is. It is unesthetic, and it too readily conducts temperature and electricity, but otherwise is close to an ideal material, except perhaps for a tendency to wear at contact points, thus shortening the teeth. (This effect is controversial and not definitely established.) Silver amalgam is formed by mixing a powder of silver (about seventy per cent), tin, copper, and zinc with pure mercury. The mix is triturated with a mortar and pestle; today this is usually done by machine rather than by hand. The mercury dissolves the metallic powder, thus forming a solution. (An amalgam is, in fact, a solution of a metal in mercury.) At this point the mass is plastic, but it will soon begin to crystallize, ultimately forming a strong, hard, solid alloy. The filling is made while the mix is in a plastic state and easily manipulated. So long as the mix is plastic, care must be taken to protect it from contamination with moisture, which would cause the filling to swell or change shape later on. The filling is carved or shaped as it is beginning to set, and it is polished one or more days later, after it is completely set. Patients are usually cautioned not to expose a new amalgam filling to strong biting pressures for a day, until it develops its full hardness.

Although a carefully conceived and well-made silver amalgam filling can be expected to last indefinitely, barring accident and assuming reasonable care by the patient, failure is nevertheless experienced quite frequently. Most failure of amalgam fillings are caused by poor dentistry, but even good work sometimes fails. If stress is placed too soon on a new and therefore brittle amalgam restoration, the result may be a hairline fracture that sometimes goes undetected for years, until continued stress dislocates a piece of the filling. Occasionally a tooth wall proves insufficiently strong to support the filling, and sooner or later the tooth itself cracks at its weak point, necessitating a new restoration. Such a break usually leaves the filling still in place and intact; this shows how strong the filling material can be. Sometimes poor oral hygiene sabotages the dentist's efforts by undermining a filled tooth with new decay, causing failure.

All the above types of failure are quite rare in the case of good restorations. The failure of *poor* restorations, on the other hand, is virtually inevitable. The notion that well-made silver fillings are impermanent is nonsense. Yet patients have told me that their dentist tried to "sell" them gold inlays to replace amalgam fillings because "silver fillings don't last." Of course, if the inlay work were of the same quality as the amalgam work, the inlays wouldn't last either.

The reasons for the failure of poorly done amalgam fillings are numerous, but all can be explained by hastiness and inattention to detail.

It is impossible to give careful attention to all these details and still complete the operation in a few minutes, as Dr. Poorwork does. It is his calculated inattention to such matters that is responsible for nearly all these failures. How does Dr. Poorwork justify his behavior? A Poorwork I know once said, "I make a filling that will hold the tooth for a few years. Isn't that worth five bucks?" I told him that holding a tooth together for a few years is indeed worth five bucks, but *only if the work is truthfully represented.* If the patient is told that the work will last only a few years, while good work will endure indefinitely, then he has a meaningful choice, and the five-dollar job, if that is what he chooses, would be worth the price. I would have no complaints about Dr. Poorwork at all if he always represented his work for what it is: substandard and inadequate. But as long as the patient thinks that one man's filling is as good as another's, as the American Dental Association leads him to believe, then he tends to select the least expensive dentist, and is deprived of a real choice.

Although amalgam, properly used, is a fine filling material, it is unsuitable for use in the front of the mouth, where the filling can be seen. Amalgam fillings often appear black against the light background of the tooth, and when they do, they are most unesthetic. Despite much research, we still do not have a really satisfactory material for front-tooth fillings. Thus far filling materials with good appearance have shown poor function, and vice versa. Routine fillings of front teeth have been known to the layman as "porcelain" fillings, though genuine porcelain is quite different from the materials actually used. True porcelain is a ceramic or clay material which must be fired in an oven at very high temperatures; obviously it cannot be shaped in the mouth, though inlays and crowns of porcelain, made outside the mouth and cemented in place, are commonly used.

The anterior filling material that has been most in favor for many years is silicate cement, presumptuously called "synthetic porcelain" by some manufacturers. Silicate cement can be made in various colors to match tooth shades, is easily manipulated, and even has a favorable coefficient of expansion. But it has poor crushing and edge strength and it therefore should not be used on a biting surface or where an edge is involved. Silicate also produces toxic reactions to the pulp of some patients and should only be used after the pulp has been carefully insulated by a protective base. The material also tends to discolor. Perhaps worst of all, it is soluble in the oral fluids of certain patients. In many mouths the most carefully prepared silicate cement fillings "wash out" after a period of time.

Faced with the shortcomings of silicate cements, dental research has been turning to newer materials. Acrylic plastics which will harden quickly have been developed; fillings made of acrylic have greater strength than the silicates, and are insoluble. On the other hand, acrylic fillings are dimensionally somewhat unstable, they are mildly toxic, they have an unfavorable coefficient of expansion, and they have a tendency to stain. Combinations of acrylic and silicate materials have been tried with unimpressive results. Newer epoxy and vinyl materials are now being tried in combinations with other plastics and inert matter. One of the more successful of the new compounds uses fine particles of glass in conjunction with plastics. Some of these materials show great promise, and though the final verdict is still not in, it may be that we will soon, and for the first time, have a fully tested, wholly satisfactory anterior filling material.

Cast gold is a much-used and respectable restorative material. Unlike gold foil, which is finely hammered pure gold placed directly in the prepared cavity, cast gold restorations are fabricated outside the mouth and are cemented into place in the prepared tooth. Fillings made in this way are called inlays. The gold inlay is an excellent restoration. It is very strong, having greater edge and crushing strength than amalgam. But, because it is made outside the mouth from impressions and models of the tooth, it cannot fit as precisely as the amalgam filling, which is formed right in the tooth itself. Moreover, the inlay must be cemented into the cavity and so needs a layer of cement between the filling and the tooth; this cement may wash out, leaving a leak in the restoration. This is the major, theoretical disadvantage of the inlay.

In the hands of a careful, skilled dentist the above difficulties can be overcome. If the tooth has been prepared with great care, and if accurate impressions have been obtained, it is possible to make an inlay that will fit with extraordinary accuracy. Because of the resulting close fit, very little cement will then be needed. In fact, a close-fitting casting does not require cement to hold it in, but primarily as a seal. After cementation, the margins of the inlay can be finished and polished so as to approximate the very close fit possible with amalgam. In the hands of the conscientious dentist, therefore, the inlay can be a superb restoration. I have seen amalgams and inlays that have been in patients' mouths for forty years, and were still in excellent condition. Good dental work does last.

Because pure gold is too soft for use in a large, cast restoration, gold inlays and crowns are cast with gold alloyed with copper, silver, and platinum, the exact components and proportion of the alloy varying with the intended use. For example, gold used for a small inlay is of a different hardness from gold used for a large crown.

Inlays, crowns, and other dental castings utilize the venerable lost-wax process. Though the method was only introduced to dentistry in 1906, the ancient historians Herodotus and Diodorus refer to bronze statues made in this manner by the Babylonians over four thousand years ago. To illustrate the lost-wax method, we will assume the construction of a medium-size inlay. The inlay is first made of wax; this can be done on a model of the prepared tooth or directly in the tooth itself. If done in the laboratory on a model, the model is first prepared from an impression of the tooth. This wax inlay, or wax pattern, must be made with the greatest care, for its duplicate in gold will be used as the finished dental restoration. The wax pattern is then invested; this means that a mold is made by pouring specially prepared plaster around it. When the plaster (investment) hardens, the wax is then burned out, leaving a mold of the pattern in plaster. Molten gold alloy is then poured into the investment mold, cooled, and cleaned with acid. The resultant castings are remarkably precise duplicates of the wax patterns.

Cast gold is used in a variety of other ways. Its use in fixed and removable dentures is covered in the chapters on prosthetics. Cast gold is also used for making gold posts, or cores. A tooth whose crown has been completely destroyed by caries or fracture can usually be restored by the use of a gold post, which is a casting made to fit into the root canal of such a tooth, with an extension to support a crown or jacket. The gold-post-and-crown restoration is occasionally called a "pivot tooth," an inaccurate term also used in the vernacular for a cantilever bridge.

The types of fillings listed above are all examples of so-called permanent fillings. Their permanence must not be taken literally, of course; though the good dentist and the patient would like them to last forever, many will not.

So-called temporary fillings, which should be used but rarely, are stop-gaps intended to be replaced by permanent restorations as soon as possible. Occasionally a tooth requires sedative medication, for example, when pulp-capping or pulpotomy procedures are being performed; in such cases the temporary filling acts as a vehicle for the medication. Temporary fillings can also be used legitimately to protect a tooth while an inlay is being made for it. Occasionally, furthermore, a dentist is confronted with widespread, serious decay and deems it important to clean out all decay in badly involved teeth at once, before making permanent restorations. These are all good, if very special, reasons for using temporaries.

On the other hand, the *routine* use of temporary fillings is bad dentistry. Routine temporaries are dear to the heart of Dr. Poorwork. One reason for this is that his patients are accustomed to paying a certain fee per visit; the temporary filling increases the number of visits, enabling the doctor to collect more for his work without the patient suspecting that the fees are, in reality, quite high. And since Poorwork rarely takes the time to remove all decay from a tooth, the sedative medication of the temporary filling, much of which will be left in the tooth under the eventually-to-be-made silver filling, will soothe the pulp and delay the inevitable toothache, so that when the toothache does finally occur, and the tooth is extracted, the patient will no longer remember that the filling was done relatively recently, and he will not connect the filling with the extraction. Furthermore, Dr. Poorwork's day is so over-booked with appointments that, even with his high-speed techniques, he often lacks the time to start and complete a filling in the same visit. On such occasions a temporary is just what he needs, even if the patient does not.

10

"Pyorrhea" -
Disease of the Gums

Pyorrhea is the single most important cause of the loss of teeth; in fact, more people wear false teeth because of the ravages of this affliction than for all other reasons combined. In the light of this statement, it may come as a shock to many that the treatment of this disease is often neglected by many dentists who should, and usually do, know better. A special tragedy of pyorrhea is that it frequently causes the loss of perfectly sound, decay-free teeth. The punch line of one of the most venerable of dental jokes, "The teeth are fine, but the gums gotta go," is unlikely to be funny to the millions who suffer from and have lost teeth because of pyorrhea.

Today the term *periodontal disease* has supplanted the obsolescent term *pyorrhea,* which literally means presence of pus; this description does not accurately define or delimit the condition. Pyorrhea also implies a specific infectious condition, which the disease is not. The more accurate term, *periodontal disease,* means disease around the tooth.

Besides the serious threat that it poses to the teeth, periodontal disease is also uncomfortable, unesthetic, and, like any chronic infectious condition, damaging to the general health and sense of well-being. It is the most prevalent cause of halitosis. In advanced cases the gums may be festering, red, spongy, tender, and oozing pus, which is swallowed with every meal. Chronic, annoying discomfort, rather than sharp pain, usually accompanies periodontal disease as it runs its long course. The mouth feels generally uncomfortable, the gums feel tight, some teeth may feel weak and tender. Forceful chewing on certain teeth may produce soreness. It is a shame that so many people go through life with such discomfort, never knowing the relief that a properly done scaling can give them until it is too late, and the teeth are lost.

Around the tooth we find what dentists call the periodontium, or supporting structures of the teeth: the alveolar part of the jawbone, the periodontal ligament, and the gingivae, or gums. These are the tissues which hold the teeth in place. Weakening and destruction of these supporting tissues results in the loosening and loss of teeth; this is the characteristic picture of periodontal disease. The alveolar bone is that part of the jawbone which immediately surrounds the teeth. Alveolar bone grows stronger in response to certain pressure, but tends to recede and be resorbed into the bloodstream in response to other, harmful, stresses. The teeth are attached to their sockets in the seemingly fickle alveolar bone by the short fibers of the periodontal ligament, also known as the periodontal membrane, though strictly speaking it is neither membrane nor ligament. The integrity of the fibers of the periodontal ligament is critical. Progressive destruction of these fibers along with the resorption of alveolar bone are always associated with advancing periodontal disease and the gradual loosening of the teeth. For further discussion of these important tissues, see especially the chapters on The Mouth, The Care of Children's Teeth, and Orthodontia.

The advertising industry has made a major effort to capitalize on the misery of those who suffer from periodontal disease, and with the usual results: It has disseminated misleading notions and wholly inaccurate information. "Bad breath," "pink toothbrush," "an army marching through your mouth," "bleeding, messy gums," "dragon in your mouth"; these are all Madison Avenue euphemisms for common symptoms of periodontal disease. The advertisements proclaim that the proper way to treat these symptoms is with the particular product being promoted; one advertisement even states that its toothpaste "gives your mouth sex appeal." The truth is, however, that the *only* way to deal with periodontal disease is with a thorough periodontal treatment by a capable dentist. Periodontal disease cannot be cured or even restrained with drugs, toothpastes, or mouthwashes. None of these preparations can do any more for a person afflicted with periodontal disease than carry away the excess pus and mask the mouth odor for a few hours; that is hardly my idea of sex appeal. It is especially dangerous that the advertised products are represented as being proper treatment for such conditions. Most adults are afflicted to some extent by periodontal disease, and the outright deceptions sponsored by the advertisers must dissuade large numbers of these people from seeking the only kind of treatment that can possibly help them.

Periodontal disease is probably the world's most widespread disease among people over the age of thirty-five. The disease and its treatment have been receiving more publicity in the last ten years than ever before. The number of periodontists, who are the specialists in the field, has increased many fold, and the body of knowledge concerning the disease has significantly increased. Yet the public is still surprisingly ignorant about the affliction. Many people still believe that so-called pyorrhea is contagious, many that it is inherited, and many that it is incurable; yet all these notions are false. Many people mistakenly attribute their gum troubles to an early case of "trench mouth" that irretrievably damaged their mouths. The proven facts and best hypotheses about periodontal disease may therefore come as a surprise to most people.

Acute pain is rarely part of the pattern of early periodontal disease; it appears only in the most advanced stages of involvement. Pericementitis, an inflammation around the root, that is detected by extreme tenderness to touch, tapping, or biting, appears when the tooth is either beyond help or can be rescued only through extensive therapy and perhaps construction of a substitute support, as by splinting it to a healthy tooth. Trench mouth, which is more fully discussed at the end of the chapter, can be very painful, but it is not necessarily part of the pattern of periodontal disease. If there were more early pain involved in periodontal disease, more people might seek treatment earlier, when it could help them more.

Periodontia, as a relatively young branch of dental science, is rife with controversy and speculation concerning the origins, prevention, and proper treatment of the disease, though most periodontists have been able to agree on certain basics. To begin with, the causes of periodontal disease are those factors which attack the integrity of the supporting tissues of the teeth; the treatment consists of measures designed to remove these causes and to bolster the defenses of the supporting tissues.

The phenomena of periodontal disease are largely attributable to the peculiar properties of the alveolar part of the jawbone, previously described. The readiness of alveolar bone to be resorbed into the bloodstream and its powers of regeneration in the young are necessary properties, which enable the baby teeth and, later, the permanent teeth to erupt through the child's jawbone. Alveolar bone in adults can still be resorbed into the bloodstream, and in response to pressures originating in periodontal disease it often is. But with age the resorption-growth pattern becomes increasingly a one-way street as the adult loses the bone-regenerative powers of the child. Thus the grown-up who is afflicted with advanced periodontal disease simply loses the alveolar bone around a tooth until there is none left to hold it in.

It is likely that the foremost cause of periodontal disease is the build-up of calculus, or tartar, which collects on the necks of the teeth and works its way down the teeth into the gum crevices. Calculus supplies mechanical, bacterial, and chemical pressure and irritation to the alveolar bone, thereby causing it to retreat. As it retreats, through resorption, the bone leaves a periodontal pocket in the gums, and this pocket becomes an unhygienic focus for more tartar formation, for the collection of mouth debris, including fermenting foods, and ultimately for active infection. These unhealthy factors all serve to promote the continuing destruction of alveolar bone. Ultimately the bone surrounding the teeth will have resorbed to such an extent that the teeth become loose and possibly painful and infected, and have to be removed. This brings us to the usual conclusion of the story of the natural teeth in unchecked periodontal disease.

The occlusion, or the way the upper and lower teeth come together as they bite, is another major factor in periodontal health and disease. An improper occlusion can generate forces on the teeth and lead to the type of stress, mentioned earlier, which causes alveolar bone resorption. Let us suppose that a tooth is slightly out of line with the other teeth in the dental arch. Whenever the jaws are brought together, as in chewing or habitually grinding the teeth, the tooth that is out of line is struck first with the full stress of the powerful masticatory action. The bone support of such a tooth is likely to break down under such a pounding. But when the occlusion is properly balanced, so that the teeth are in good alignment, the stresses resulting from mastication are well distributed throughout the mouth, and actually tend to strengthen the alveolar bone, rather than to cause its resorption. These examples of what happens under conditions of good and bad occlusion are grossly oversimplified, but they do give a reasonably accurate picture of the role of occlusion in the health of the mouth.

A dental arch deformed as the result of a missing, unreplaced tooth has been seriously weakened, and is very likely to show periodontal disorders in the future. A lost tooth, unless and until it is replaced, leaves a space in the mouth. As a rule, the other teeth presently begin to shift position, as described in the chapter entitled "Concerning Extractions." Such shifts must result in a weakening and distortion of the dental arches, poor occlusion, and an increased vulnerability to decay. The teeth, having shifted, now present areas where food can get caught, making the mouth more difficult to clean and highly susceptible to future disease.

Poor dental restorations are a very common cause

of periodontal disease. Restorations with poor margins irritate the gums, while restorations that do not assure good occlusion can cause all the periodontal consequences of poor occlusion, including temporomandibular disorders. Other restorations, that fail to reestablish the proper points of contact between the teeth, can result in food-trap areas and, before long, may damage the periodontium. It should be obvious, therefore, that before a dentist makes any dental restoration, he owes it to his patient to consider carefully what the periodontal consequences of the work will be.

Habits play an important role in periodontal disease. The tension-induced habit of grinding the teeth is discussed later. Any habit that causes repeated muscular pressure against teeth can be damaging to their periodontal health. The tongue may settle habitually between two teeth, and exert pressure on them, or the lips may perform habitual sucking or smacking motions; such persistent habits are capable of weakening the teeth that are exposed to them. Habitual ways of holding a pipe, cigar, or cigarette, of playing a wind instrument, of holding nails or safety pins in the teeth, of chewing fingernails, are all potential causes of periodontal damage. Even some habits of speech, eating, and facial expression can weaken the supporting structure of one or more teeth. The treatment for such habits *includes their diagnosis* (because merely to understand them may help the patient to bring them under control), analysis, and, if need be, systematic correction by the cooperative efforts of dentist and patient.

Systemic disorders, which relate to the condition of the body as a whole, are also capable of influencing the health of the periodontium. Nutritional deficiencies, debilitating and degenerative diseases, metabolic disorders, even mental health—all can play a part. But, compared to the major factors already discussed, and compared to habits of oral hygiene, the systemic disorders play a relatively minor role.

The habits of oral hygiene are a critical factor. The most elaborate treatment of the disease cannot succeed unless the patient attends conscientiously to his oral hygiene. Neglect not only increases the likelihood of tooth decay, but also contributes to the build-up of calculus, plaque, materia alba, and a generalized filthy condition which, coupled with the weakening of the gums by calculus and other irritants, can lead to chronic inflammation and infection, itself a factor in the disease. Dental plaque is a conglomerate of food debris and microorganisms associated with decay and periodontal destruction. Materia alba (literally, "white stuff") is a residue of soft, partially digested food that is undoubtedly a factor in plaque production. Materia alba and plaque comprise a kind of unesthetic mouth slime that provides a continual source of chemical irritation to the gingivae and bone. Careful oral hygiene should all but eliminate these local irritants. To check the efficiency of your oral hygiene, run a fingernail over the face of a front tooth and see what you scrape up. If you discover under the nail some whitish, slimy material, then your oral hygiene is inadequate. If the fingernail scrapes up nothing, don't congratulate yourself until trying the same test on a more remote surface of a back tooth. If you are with the great majority of people, your oral hygiene practices could be much improved.

Diet is an important part of the story of periodontal disease only if there is inadequate oral hygiene. Diets high in carbohydrates, when combined with poor oral hygiene, leave film, debris, and plaque on the teeth and around the gums. This situation, which also favors dental decay, accelerates the formation of calculus and promotes bacterial irritation, and thus can lead to the destruction of bone. But diet may also have an opposite effect. A person who customarily eats coarse, heavy-crusted, chewy breads and raw vegetables is likely to have a healthy periodontal situation. The raw vegetables are examples of "detergent" foods which actually help clean the mouth, and the heavy chewing gives the bone additional healthy exercise, in favorable directions, which usually results in stronger, disease-resistant bone.

The question of the proper treatment of periodontal disease is far from being settled. There is controversy over occlusion, surgery, and even methods of brushing. While the following discussion of treatments concentrates on the mainstream of current thought, it also gives some attention to alternative treatments on which there is less agreement.

There is no controversy about the removal of calculus, or tartar. Calculus almost invariably destroys tissue, and it must be removed. Removal is accomplished by procedures called scaling or curettage, the latter term often being used to indicated a very deep scaling, with the scraping and removal of sick tissue. Scalers and curettes, the instruments used in this work, are small, sharp knives which scrape clean the root surfaces of the teeth. Gross supragingival calculus, that can be seen above the gum line, is relatively easy to remove. Calculus that is deep under the gums is more difficult. Scalers and curettes are manipulated beneath the gums right down to the level of greatest pocket depth, practically to the bone. The scraping, that removes the calculus, is done upwards and with great care, because misuse of the instruments may damage the tissues and fail to remove some of the calculus. The treatment can be effective only when all the calculus is removed. This is painstaking, tedious work;

like other dental procedures, *it takes time*. Any good dentist or periodontist may spend many hours, spread over several visits, just removing the calculus from one patient's mouth.

The Cavitron is another instrument which has been used for calculus and stain removal. This instrument does its work through supersonic vibrations, and, up to a point, it does a creditable job. Most periodontists feel that the instrument cannot remove all traces of deep, subgingival calculus. This is why those who use the Cavitron usually complete the job with scalers and curettes.

It is universally agreed that improper occlusion can be deadly to the health of the periodontium. An occlusal prematurity is a tooth surface which comes into contact with its opposing tooth before the rest of the other teeth come into contact. A "high" tooth takes quite a beating, bearing, as it must, the entire thrust of the biting force before the other teeth meet to take their share. One of the simplest ways to discover an occlusal prematurity is with the use of articulating paper, a strip of waxed carbon paper inserted between the teeth, that leaves a colored mark on the high spot of a tooth when the patient bites down on it. A simple treatment for a high spot is to grind it down a bit, eliminating the interfering high area of the tooth and thus bringing the tooth back into line. It is not always so easy. Complex jaw movements in various excursions, or chewing motions from side to side, often make analysis and correction quite difficult.

Once the diagnosis of traumatic occlusion is made, the dentist begins to take steps to correct occlusal defects, in so far as they may be remediable. To this end he may reshape certain teeth by grinding them so as to develop a better balance of masticatory stresses; he may build up other teeth, with crowns; and he may replace missing teeth. Elaborate procedures such as these are often undertaken in close consultation with a periodonist.

Bruxism and Bruxomania

Many dentists feel that the destructive effects of poor occlusion may occur less during eating and chewing than during habitual grinding. It is surprising how many people give vent to their tensions by clenching or grinding the teeth. Grinding may occur while the patient is awake or asleep. The dental term for the habit of teeth-grinding during waking hours is bruxomania; its more common, sleepytime counterpart is called bruxism. Grinding can produce enormous pressures, particularly on teeth that are out of line, and these pressures may cause rapid resorption of bone. Sometimes a poorly thought-out or badly executed restoration (filling, crown, bridge, or partial denture) has changed the occlusion and led to new patterns of habitual grinding which have rapidly destroyed the alveolar bone support of some teeth. I have seen cases in which a change of grinding habits had, within a few months, completely destroyed the bone around certain teeth and had virtually knocked them out of the mouth. Any restoration that alters the bite even slightly runs the risk of setting up such ruinous patterns of grinding. It is partly because of this danger that every dentist worth his salt takes however much time is needed to restore carefully a proper, functional occlusion in each restoration that involves a biting surface.

Dentists and periodontists sometimes use a night-guard to prevent the damage caused by severe bruxism. A night-guard usually consists of a plastic, horseshoe-shaped shell that fits over the upper teeth and is worn at night. The idea is to relieve the afflicted teeth of the dangerous concentration of pressure by distributing the force of the grinding more evenly over the dentition. In some cases the night-guard also helps to cure the bruxist of his habit by changing the "feel" of the mouth.

Grinding when awake can be more of a problem, since it is inconvenient to use a night-guard during waking hours. In severe cases of bruxomania the aim is to keep the patient continuously aware of the habit, in the hope that he may thereby learn to control it. All sorts of treatments have been tried, including suggestion, hypnotism, and even psychotherapy.

One of the most frustrating problems in dentistry involves the temporomandibular articulation. This is the scientific name of the complex hinge-type joint located just in front of the middle part of the ear; if you place a finger at that area and move the lower jaw, you will be able to feel the lower jaw as it moves in the socket of the upper jaw. A malfunction of this joint can produce annoying and hard-to-diagnose symptoms. The joint itself may ache. Persistant headaches may radiate from the joint to the top of the head, or localize at the top of the head. The patient may hear "clicking" sounds, apparently from the inside of the head. These symptoms may be very depressing; people afflicted with persistent non-diagnosed pain are rarely good company.

The effect of tension and stress, magnified by improper occlusion, has been established as the major factor in disturbances of the temporomandibular joint. Very often, restoration of the mouth to proper occlusion dramatically relieves all symptoms. Here is how this works in theory. The lower jaw is movable, the upper jaw is not. The workings of the temporomandibular joint depend in part on how the teeth meet during the movements of chewing and grinding food. Also most significant are the positions the jaws may take under conditions of bruxism and bruxomania, when the teeth may be grinding in an awkward position or the jaws may be locked under tension in an eccentric position. Malocclusion or awkward patterns of bruxism may place the jaws in a strained position at the temporomandibular joint, resulting in pain, possibly from stretched ligaments, muscles, or tendons, or perhaps from an arthritic involvement resulting from the strain. It is as if one persisted in straining an elbow while it is in some awkward position. Many baseball pitchers and tennis players will confirm that, under just such persistent strain, the elbow may become painful.

The treatment of these cases by correcting the bite can be a very complicated matter, although in some cases it can be simply achieved. Elaborate techniques of great complexity and sophistication, many of them controversial, have been developed for diagnosis and treatment. The crucial question again is, What, exactly, is the proper occlusion for the particular patient? The results of the work now being done in this field are somewhat encouraging, and it is fair to say that people suffering from the depressing effects of temporomandibular joint malfunction now have a better chance of obtaining relief than ever before, and that the chances are still improving.

Splinting and Surgery

Some advanced cases of periodontal disease are best treated surgically. If there are pockets where bone has been resorbed deep along the root of a tooth, or between the roots of multirooted teeth, surgery is often performed in an attempt to remove unhealthy tissue, clean out the pocket, and reshape the bone so as to leave a healthier, hygienic periodontium, and get a healed, healthy gum snuggling against a root that is more easily kept clean. The indications for periodontal surgery are highly controversial, and so are its methods. Some periodontists, for example, prefer to rely almost entirely upon such conservative measures as scaling, curettage, occlusal adjustments, and meticulous oral hygiene. But today the pendulum is swinging the other way, and most periodontists are quite willing to perform surgery. There are advocates of each of a number of different surgical techniques, including electrosurgery, in which the gum is trimmed off electrically, and cryosurgery, in which the gum is frozen off by an electrical freezing instrument. Many dentists and periodontists are partial to more conventional surgery, in which the gum is cut, with scalpels, to the level of the pocket. There are also ingenious and, in the author's opinion, sensible methods of removing unhealthy tissue inside the gum with scalpels and curettes, and then suturing the gum back to its original position. Whatever the best techniques may be, it is clear that excellent results are often obtained through surgery. However, the readiness of some periodontists to perform these procedures may possibly reflect, in addition to a commendable zeal to cure the patient, a desire to justify the high fee.

A tooth or teeth seriously weakened by loss of alveolar bone can in many cases be bolstered by splinting to stronger, adjacent teeth. Many types of splints are used; the exact choice depends upon individual requirements. Temporary splints may be made of wire alone, or of wire reinforced with plastic. Splints that are meant to last indefinitely are made with crowns, pin-castings, and other expensive procedures. Careful use of splinting methods, coupled with thorough treatment, has

saved teeth that, not so long ago, would have been condemned as hopeless.

Poorwork and Periodontia

When it comes to periodontia, Dr. Poorwork is as
effective in destroying mouths as he is in anything else
he does. For one thing, his hasty, ill-conceived, and
poorly executed restorations are in themselves often
prime causes of periodontal destruction. Furthermore,
it is the duty of the general practitioner to see that
the patient who needs periodontal care receives it.
Poorwork should either do the work himself or inform
the patient of the condition and refer him to a periodontist. But he does neither, and again the reasons
are economic.

The bulk of Dr. Poorwork's dental work has always
been limited to what his patients will readily accept
and pay for at rates that return him a healthy profit.
He is not too happy about periodontal treatment,
which takes too much time, and for which his patients
are not accustomed to paying. Certainly he recognizes
"pyorrhea" and the discomfort it causes. He is prepared to ease discomfort with various chemical palliative treatments, such as peroxide mouthwashes,
applications of gentian violet, and, in some cases, even
antibiotic therapy; these are all treatments which
may take him five minutes or less. His idea of routine
periodontal care consists of the "cleaning," a process
that takes just a few minutes as he scrapes off a little
tartar and polishes the teeth, especially the front ones,
with some pumice paste. His patients accept this work
at a low fee, but are too ill-informed to accept a high
fee for a thorough scaling, which may take hours.

Peroxide usually reduces the inflammation and pain
of an acute flare-up of gingivitis. Gentian violet, the

dark purple dye so often used for gingivitis, is useless; warm water rinses are much more effective. In the raging forms of mouth infection, discussed below, Dr. Poorwork sometimes resorts to penicillin or other antibiotics; some Poorworks even use antibiotics for milder infections, though the practice is condemned by responsible authorities. Some of these methods provide temporary relief, but none can control the relentless bone destruction caused by the many factors of periodontal disease, not one of which is removed by chemical therapy. At their best, chemical treatments simply mask the disease and its occasional acute flare-ups until irrevocable damage has been done, and the teeth have become painful. Then Dr. Poorwork begins to remove teeth and make a series of cheap relacement appliances which, over the years, are in turn discarded to make way for full dentures. His patients, having been taught that pyorrhea is incurable, accept their fate quietly.

A patient of Dr. Goodwork, on the other hand, is given enough information to make a choice. But too many patients, having been weaned on Dr. Poorwork, have said to Dr. Goodwork's prescription for periodontal care: "What! Fifty dollars (or more) for a cleaning!" And so, suspecting that Goodwork's periodontal treatment is just a fancy, expensive cleaning, the patient goes back to Dr. Poorwork—and to years of advancing periodontal disease.

Trench Mouth

The condition known by the colorful term *trench* mouth is also called Vincent's disease and, more accurately, ANUG, which stands for acute necrotizing ulcerative gingivitis. ANUG is a painful, infectious flare-up of an unclean mouth. It is not found in mouths that have consistently had the benefit of good oral hygiene, and therefore it cannot be considered to be contagious, except, perhaps, under conditions of universal poor oral hygiene, as in the trenches in World War I. Trench mouth should not be confused with periodontal disease, though mouth tissues that have been weakened by incipient periodontal disease are more susceptible to an attack of trench mouth. Periodontal disease can run its course without an episode of ANUG, and conversely, ANUG is often seen in filthy mouths of young people not yet affected by periodontal disease. In my own practice I have never observed a case of ANUG in a mouth accustomed to good oral hygiene.

Although a full-blown case of ANUG is most annoying, and can even be extremely painful, its treatment is relatively simple. It consists of cleaning up the mouth and putting the patient on a regimen of warm water rinses and good oral hygiene. Scaling should be done as soon as the gum condition allows. The *limited* use of an oxygenating mouthwash, such as peroxide, is often helpful in reducing initial inflammation. I believe that antibiotics should not be used except in otherwise uncontrollable cases.

While examining patients suffering from advanced periodontal disease I have often heard statements like this: "I had trench mouth when I was young, and from then on my gums were ruined." The intended implication, that it was the trench mouth that caused persistent periodontal disease, puts the situation entirely out of focus. The statement is based on a series of misconceptions. Though the initial episode of acute gingivitis was probably the first sign of trouble that the patient noticed, it was poor oral hygiene that brought on the trench mouth, and it was poor oral hygiene, very probably compounded by dental neglect, over the years, that was responsible for the continued periodontal destruction. It is very likely that the patient's first gingival flare-up was improperly treated, perhaps with useless gentian violet or a mouthwash. It is improbable that such treatment was followed up with scalings and other necessary periodontal work. The result, of course, was that the periodontal condition progressively worsened. Obviously, therefore, it is completely wrong to blame the "ruined gums" on an early case of trench mouth.

Summary: Is Periodontal Disease Curable?

The good dentist regularly checks the periodontal condition of his patients. He uses X-rays to detect bone damage, and clinical examination to discover the condition of the gums (whether pockets have formed, and so on) and occlusal problems. Routine preventive periodontal care includes thorough scalings at regular intervals, from every three months to once a year, depending on the patient. It is not normal for the gums to bleed when they are being brushed; bleeding usually means that a scaling is overdue. If your gums bleed frequently, and your dentist treats the condition with a perfunctory "cleaning" and mouthwashes, it may be time to look for another dentist.

Periodontal disease is neither incurable nor completely curable. Bone destroyed by the disease cannot be restored, though heavy research, some of it promising, is being done on this critical problem. The idea in back of periodontal treatment is to arrest the disease and thus to prevent further destruction. Dramatic successes have been achieved, even in what seemed to be nearly hopeless cases. Both the experience of modern practice and the weight of experimental evidence have led me to believe that, if preventive care is started early enough, by both the dentist and his patient, almost no one now needs to lose teeth because of so-called pyorrhea.

11

The Truth About Toothpaste and Oral Hygiene

The good dentist is trained and ready to treat a wide variety of mouth disorders: Caries, malocclusion, missing teeth, trauma, infectious and degenerative disease, and others. In most cases, furthermore, he can achieve remarkably successful results, *provided he has the patient's full cooperation.* There is a catch in those italicized words, because the dentist, by himself, is nearly helpless when it comes to the single most important cause of dental disease. That cause is poor oral hygiene; the very best work the dentist can do may not succeed in a mouth not kept meticulously clean. Because he is aware of this problem, the modern dentist is willing to spend as much time as is necessary to teach patients the principles and methods of home care.

Some idea of the importance of oral hygiene has seeped through to the public through the efforts of Madison Avenue. Relying on its most hallowed principle, that a little knowledge is a profitable thing, the advertising industry has enriched itself and some of its clients by building up and exploiting the public's vague fears about the dangers of poor oral hygiene. Yet, after years of watching television commercials for dental products, I cannot recall a single advertisement which, either directly or by implication, did not seek to mislead the viewer. Watching TV for less than an hour last night, I saw two toothpaste commercials and one for a mouthwash; all three spouted misinformation and false claims. The social and intellectual climate created by such encouragement of misunderstanding and such pandering to ignorance makes it doubly difficult for the dentist to set his patients straight on the all-important matters of oral hygiene. Here, to clear the air before we go any farther, are the refutations of some of the more dangerously false ideas spread by the makers of toothpastes and other preparations:

1. The natural color of adult teeth is *not* white, and it is harmful to teeth to try to scrub them until they get white. Harsh scouring, to whiten teeth, with the aid of one of the so-called whitening abrasive toothpastes, can cause severe damage to the dentition. The natural color of a tooth is yellowish, ranging from a gray-yellow to a light reddish-yellow. This color range holds for all races of mankind: White, black, yellow, and others. Of course, teeth do look lighter against the background of a naturally dark complexion, and the smile of even a fair-skinned person looks brighter when he has a deep tan.

2. It is the toothbrush, not the dentifrice, that does the important work when the teeth are brushed. The choice of toothpaste or tooth powder probably makes little difference, so long as it is not

harmful, as by being too abrasive. But gentle dentifrices *are* helpful in that their detergents, mild scouring abrasives, and foaming agents help to carry off the debris dislodged by the brush.

3. No mouthwash, toothpaste, or lozenge can cure halitosis, and commercial mouthwashes are dangerous if used consistently. It is true that most cases of what the hucksters coyly call bad breath are caused by conditions in the mouth; but the most a mouthwash or other preparation can do for such a condition is to mask just one of its effects, the foul breath and bad taste, very briefly. Meanwhile the condition which causes the unpleasant mouth odor freely attacks the gums behind the masking counter-odor of the mouth rinse, or whatever it is. Any commercial mouthwash, if used consistently, may destroy the natural chemical and bacteriological balance of the mouth. New, unforeseen difficulties may result; and the old difficulty, for which the mouthwash was unwisely used, is likely to become worse than ever.

4. Nearly all commercial products sold to wearers of dentures are useless or worse—usually worse. This includes items sold in drug stores, chain food stores, and by mail. For further information on this point, and on the hygiene and care of removable false teeth, see the chapter on "Dentures: Hygiene and Hazards.

The direct purpose of oral hygiene is to remove the dirt, or oral debris, from the mouth. Oral debris has just one source, and that is food. As we eat, small fragments of unswallowed food collect between the teeth, along the edges of the gums, and elsewhere in the mouth. In the chemical and bacterial environment of the mouth these food residues soon begin to ferment, while some are partially digested by the saliva. It is under these oral conditions that the food that gets stuck in the mouth, instead of being swallowed, contributes to the formation of materia alba, dental plaque, and calculus, or tartar, and leads in this way to tooth decay and periodontal disease. Removing food residues from the mouth promptly after eating reduces these unpleasant results to a minimum, but this is easier said than done. While there is a direct correlation between oral-hygiene efforts and a reduction in oral disease, the methods of oral hygiene, even when applied assiduously, are not always completely effective.

Food residues tend to collect at the gingival sulcus, or gum-edge, that part of the gum where tooth meets gum, and in other hard-to-reach areas of the mouth, such as the occlusal grooves on the biting surfaces of back teeth and areas between teeth where food may tend to wedge, and where the toothbrush reaches only with difficulty. These areas, not surprisingly, are the very locations where decay most commonly forms; they should be given most careful attention during brushing.

The mouth has a tendency to keep itself clean, though the effect varies with the individual. Some mouths are very easy to keep clean, and usually have little dental trouble; others are very difficult to keep clean, and tend to resist the best efforts of oral hygiene. The saliva washes the mouth. The tongue and the other muscles of the mouth, lips, and cheek tend to cleanse the oral cavity. The viscosity and flow of a given person's saliva, the shape and action of his mouth tissues, and his habits all bear on the ease or difficulty of keeping his particular mouth clean. Consequently, some people can maintain excellent oral hygiene with relatively little effort, while others have to take careful measures after every meal and even every snack. But whether the mouth is easy or difficult to keep clean, anyone who expects to keep his mouth healthy has to take the time necessary to learn the methods of good home care, and must also take as much time as is needed, each day, to maintain proper oral hygiene.

Though the teeth need to be brushed, it has been said with a good bit of truth that it is even more important to brush the gums, in order to remove food debris from the gum-edge area. Many cavities start here, and this is where calculus begins to form. Methods of brushing may vary. One popular and effective method utilizes a short-headed brush with extra-hard bristles. The brush is manipulated carefully from gum to tooth, always from gum to tooth, except on the biting surfaces, which are scrubbed with vigor. Another method utilizes a very soft brush which is vibrated right into the gingival sulci. The electric toothbrushes, getting more popular, in essence utilize this soft-brush method. Properly designed electric toothbrushes, carefully used, can do an excellent job, though some authorities oppose them on the ground that they are potentially harmful; the author is in favor of most kinds. Either method gives good results if enough time and care are taken to cover *every surface of every* tooth, and the surrounding gums. It takes some degree of dexterity to accomplish this. An advantage of the electric toothbrush is that less skill, and hence less practice, is needed to achieve the desired result. The best way to learn proper toothbrushing methods is to ask your dentist to demonstrate them. Most good dentists, realizing the critical importance of oral hygiene, are set up to demonstrate oral hygiene methods, and are always glad to do so.

The oral hygiene of young children presents special problems. The major difficulty is that they lack the dexterity to brush their teeth effectively. Furthermore, the eating habits of the typical child are such that he is likely to have food residues in his mouth much of the time. See the chapter on Dental Decay for a further discussion of this important subject.

Some authorities have expressed concern that the milk given to bottle-fed infants may help to produce caries. It is true that milk sweetened by sugars or honey or supplemented with carbohydrate additives can have a powerful decay-producing effect on infants' teeth. But milk to which no sugar, chocolate, or starches have been added has no caries-producing effect; on the contrary, pure milk has been found to somewhat inhibit decay.

The child should receive instructions in brushing at a very early age, and every day he should be given an opportunity to brush his own teeth; this will help to build good oral-hygiene habits. But as long as he is young he cannot be expected to manipulate the brush properly. Therefore a parent must also brush the child's teeth each day, to remove plaque, film, and food debris.

Timing is a critical factor in oral hygiene. The purpose is, of course, to remove oral debris from the mouth. Since the *only* source of oral debris is food, it is logical to use oral-hygiene techniques *after* eating; it is absurd to brush first, eat with a clean mouth, and then leave the mouth filthy. In my experience, it seems that many people who believe they exercise careful oral hygiene make the serious mistake of brushing only before breakfast and before going to sleep. Most of their oral-hygiene efforts are wasted; their mouths are unclean for perhaps sixteen hours each day, and they are clean for only the amount of time they are abed.

There are many adjuncts to the toothbrush which may improve one's oral hygiene. A simple, common, and effective, though underrated, technique involves the use of a glass of water. Thorough, forceful rinsing of the mouth after brushing is a must. Caries-prone individuals can also be helped considerably by strong rinsing with water after snacks or drinks; of course brushing, if possible, is even better. Ordinary water is also, by all odds, the best mouthwash. Dental floss, dental tapes, and toothpicks are the best-known mechanical allies of the toothbrush. Dental floss is strong thread which is passed between two adjoining teeth to remove debris wedged between them; dental floss is also helpful in cleaning the edges of the gums between the teeth. Dental tapes are used much like dental floss; I prefer floss. The toothpick can be handy in removing an annoyingly wedged piece of food, but the toothpick lends itself to misuse; dental floss is safer and more effective. Stim-U-Dents are proprietary toothpicks of very sophisticated design. Some dentists and periodontists recommend them routinely for therapeutic home care. The Pick-A-Dent is a proprietary, double-ended, soft plastic toothpick; one end has a point, like that of an ordinary toothpick, while the other end is shaped like a Stim-U-Dent. If carried around, it will occasionally come in handy. Zon is a proprietary, flexible plastic needle, that can be threaded with dental floss, enabling one to get the floss into otherwise inaccessible areas—underneath the false teeth of fixed bridgework, for example.

The Water Pik, also a proprietary product, represents a significant advance in oral-hygiene technology. The Water Pik, and each of its host of imitators, is a pumping device with a small, easily directed plastic nozzle that delivers a strong, pulsating stream of water to spaces between the teeth. The device can clean out an enormous amount of debris which the toothbrush, in the hands of the average person, never reaches. It is especially useful in mouths with extensive fixed bridge-work. Though the Water Pik has not yet been in use long enough for the dental profession to reach a definite, unanimous conclusion, it does seem likely that the device will come to be regarded as an important part of the oral-hygiene apparatus of very many people. But some precautions must be observed. The indiscriminate use of the Water Pik may do harm in mouths afflicted with advanced, untreated periodontal disease. The device may also hasten the dissolution of the cement seal of poorly made crowns and inlays having inaccurate margins; this effect does not occur with well-made restorations having sound margins. All in all, it is best to use the Water Pik under the guidance of a good dentist.

The effects of toothpastes and mouthwashes can be understood only in relation to the natural chemistry of the mouth. The chief factor here is the saliva, which is discussed more fully in the chapter entitled On the Mouth. Saliva comes from the salivary glands. (As an aside, it should be mentioned that a duct from one of these glands occasionally becomes blocked by calcification. This leads to an annoying and sometimes painful swelling of the gland, which can be treated by removing the stone blocking the duct.) The importance of the saliva in maintaining good oral hygiene could not conceivably be overestimated. Though the mouth is on a par with the anus as a center for microorganisms —over eighty known varieties are commonly domiciled in the mouth—these organisms, always under the influence of the saliva, tend to keep each other in balance and under control, so that they do not themselves cause any harmful infection.

Suppose that into this unique natural environment we now introduce a strong chemical that kills off a good many of the microorganisms normally found in the mouth. A not-unlikely result is that the surviving types of microorganisms will proliferate now that their natural enemies have been killed off by the chemical. The consequent serious imbalance in the oral population can lead to trouble; in fact, it often does. This is exactly what happens when a chemical mouthwash is used frequently. Just for example, continuous use of any peroxide mouthwash to "treat" bleeding gums kills some of the varieties of bacteria in the mouth. The result is the proliferation of certain varieties of microfungi that were previously kept in check by the killed bacteria. This may lead to an ugly fungus infection descriptively called black, hairy tongue. If caught early, black, hairy tongue will clear up promptly, once the peroxide mouthwash is discontinued.

The use of any medicated mouthwash should be reserved for specific, rare conditions, and should not be prolonged. Furthermore, mouthwashes should not be used at all except as directed by a dentist. Yet millions of Americans, prodded by persistent advertising, do use mouthwashes habitually. In some of these people the resulting oral environment has changed to accommodate the chemistry of the mouthwash, and in some cases even to *rely* on it. Thus a new, artificial chemical and microbiological balance is established that, compared with nature's balance, is extremely precarious, and may easily be upset. By far the best mouthwash is ordinary water, and the best therapeutic mouthwash for most infectious conditions is hot salt water. People who have, in a sense, become addicted to the taste of a mouthwash, and who will make the effort, will find they can easily adjust to the taste of water.

How about that "horrible morning taste" in the mouth, which many people like to dispel with brushing before breakfast? Again, this is a matter of habit. The healthy mouth quickly accommodates to the taste of a water rinse before breakfast, and a brushing afterwards, and stays much healthier. Mouths with genuinely foul tastes, which water may not dispel, probably suffer from periodontal disease, and should receive treatment.

Toothpastes with extremely strong and even irritating flavors have, for some reason, become popular lately. These strong flavors have absolutely nothing to do with oral hygiene, and they are actually dangerous in that they effectively mask the symptoms of oral disease and may therefore cause serious delays in seeking treatment. Yet strong-flavored toothpastes are universally peddled by Madison Avenue with the false implication that they are somehow more effective. This is just another example of the public-be-damned, let's-sell-some-toothpaste attitude of the advertising industry.

Many extravagantly advertised chemical additives have been used in toothpastes. Over the last fifteen years these have included carbamide (urea), chlorophyll, hexachlorophene, sodium lauryl sulphate, and various forms of fluoride. Much of what has been called research has gone into demonstrating the superiority of toothpastes containing these additives. It must be puzzling to some people to hear one TV commercial proclaim that little Johnny's group had thirty-seven per cent fewer cavities because they used toothpaste A, and then to find out from another commercial that Billy's group had thirty-nine per cent fewer cavities because *they* used toothpaste B. Those who are sophisticated in the ways of big business and Madison Avenue may not be surprised to learn that "research" that "proves" that Colgate is superior is, curiously enough, sponsored by Colgate, while "research" demonstrating the superiority of Crest has been paid for by the makers of Crest. And it may not be surprising to learn, further-more, that subsequent independent research has not confirmed the earlier reports sponsored by the adver-tisers.

A close look at some of this "research" is revealing. As an example, let us examine some features of a rela-tively simple study designed to test an anti-caries prod-uct. A number of children, six to eleven years of age, were split into two groups. One group, the control, brushed their teeth *once only,* under supervision, with a tooth-cleaning paste. The experimental group brushed their teeth *once only* also, and also under supervision, with the same tooth-cleaning paste, but to which the anti-caries ingredient had been added. The report claimed that after one year, as a result of this solitary test brushing, the experimental group had acquired no less than forty per cent fewer caries than the control group. This is an astonishing result, which would ap-pear to be of great scientific significance—until we examine the report more closely.

In any scientific study it is essential that the con-trol and experimental groups be as nearly identical as possible and that every effort be made to eliminate variables that might affect the result. But in this study the control group, *presumably* selected to be as much like the experimental group as possible, *actually* start-ed with twenty-two per cent more decayed teeth than the experimental group. The control group was there-fore *considerably* more caries-active than the experi-mental group. In any study of caries it is inexcusable to select as a control group individuals who are demon-strably so much more susceptible to caries than the experimental group. Moreover, the handling of the statistical conclusions in the report is also open to ques-tion (though we need not go into the details here). With these critical considerations the claimed reduction of caries no longer seems impressive, if indeed it means anything at all.

A critical examination of this type of dental "research" leaves too many unanswered questions, which raise grave doubts about the usefulness and realism of the published results. The dental histories and experience of the members of the control and experimental groups; oral-hygiene instruction, or lack of it, given to the two groups; tooth-brushing supervision, or lack of it, given to the two groups; the socio-economic backgrounds of the two groups; the possibilities of caries-inducing diet: These are all examples of factors that must be considered in any study of caries. But such consideration is missing from most of the studies I have seen. When little Johnny's group has thirty-one per cent fewer cavities, is it because his group used the magic ingredient, or because their oral hygiene was carefully supervised? When one toothpaste company publishes a dramatic decrease in cavities attributed to their current new ingredient, and then a manufacturer of a toothpaste *not using this ingredient* publishes a study showing equivalent results, the only reasonable conclusion to draw is that better oral hygiene, and not dramatic ingredients, are the answer.

Carbamide (urea) was used about ten years ago as a toothpaste additive, but did not find favor and is hardly used any more, possibly because people consider a uric acid derivative unesthetic for mouth use. Chlorophyll has never been shown to have any value of any sort whatever, though it does, at least, make a nice green color. Hexachlorophene is simply a detergent. Sodium lauryl sulphate and fluoride compounds are supposed to have specific anticarious properties. In the author's opinion this has not been clearly established for either type of compound, though the fluorides probably do some good. The action of fluoride, *when taken internally,* is well known; taken by children, with their water, it greatly increases the caries-resistance of the teeth. The evidence of its effectiveness when applied directly to the teeth is much less impressive. However, I do not hesitate to recommend any of the fluoride toothpastes; they cannot do any harm, and they may do some good.

A full discussion of the controversy concerning fluoridation of the water supply is outside the scope of this book. Suffice it to say here that fluoridation is by far the most extensively studied and documented scientific program in history. Fluoridation of public drinking water reduces decay by fifty to seventy per cent. And of some eighty million Americans and millions of other people around the world drinking fluoridated water over the past twenty five years there has not been one authenticated case of a person who has been harmed by it.

Agents other than conventional commercial toothpastes have been used as dentifrices. Among these are salt, bicarbonate of soda, soaps, pumice, and plain water. Conventional, mild toothpastes assist the brush in removing stains from the teeth; they do a somewhat better job than plain water. Salt and bicarbonate of soda are much too abrasive to be used as dentifrices. Soaps have an unpleasant taste. Though the dentist uses flour of pumice for polishing and "cleanings," plain pumice is much too abrasive. Flour of pumice is extremely finely milled pumice stone, which comes from volcanic lava. While acceptable for occasional use, even fine flour of pumice is much too abrasive for regular use in the mouth. There are cases on record of patients who, having heard the dentist say he used pumice to clean their teeth, went to a hardware store and bought regular pumice, which is much coarser than flour of pumice, and brushed their teeth with it. In some cases the pumice wore the teeth down to small stumps. Any mild, conventional toothpaste, perhaps with fluoride, is the best and safest dentifrice to use. It doesn't make much difference which one you pick, because, as we have said, it's the toothbrush that does nearly all the work.

The late TV mystery fades out at a moment critical to the plot. The scene changes; the camera pans a lovely beach landscape and moves in to a close-up of a worried girl. Not until she speaks do you realize you have left Hollywood for Madison Avenue. This pretty young lady, face creased with anxiety, is confiding to her friend about her romantic difficulties with the newly-met male eligible of her choice. "Why," she says, "he acts aloof; almost as if I had *(agonized pause)* BAD BREATH!" The dread possibility evokes from this girl a look of such poignant horror that one knows she would receive a diagnosis of terminal cancer with relative equanimity. Her friend, wise in the ways of the cosmetic counter, has the reassuring answer: "Don't worry, XYZ Mouthwash keeps breath fresh and clean for hours!" The next scene shows our heroine, fully recovered from her recent anxiety attack, being complimented by her friend, who is saying, with a knowing smile, "I see everything is just swell." "Yes", replies ex-anxious, "thanks to you, and XYZ Mouthwash." So saying, she and young eligible, arm in arm, head off toward the sunset-illumined hills—perhaps to open their own advertising agency and bring similar happiness to others. Before the knowledgeable viewer becomes sufficiently infuriated at the absurd implications and even the downright *lie* of the whole commercial to do something about it—send a telegram to a congressman, threaten the manufacturer, picket the advertising agency, or maybe just kick his own TV—he is back at the movies, in a gloomy mansion with a young lady about to be murdered. The male lead gets close to her whenever he can—as close as possible—so you know *she* doesn't have bad breath.

I have said it before, but it is worth repeating: Mouthwashes, toothpastes, and so on, cannot conceivably cure any type of halitosis, despite the solemn affirmations of the hucksters. What the proprietary products *will* do is to mask the taste, odors, and discomfort of the mouth condition for a brief period of time. It is like putting perfume on garbage and living with it instead of making an effort to remove the garbage; this can be particularly poignant when the garbage is in one's own mouth. The astringent and anesthetic action of the chemical agents in these preparations may give a diseased, foul-smelling mouth a temporary feeling of well-being, which is dangerous if the person is thereby dissuaded from seeking proper treatment. Untreated, the destructive periodontal condition will continue until crippling damage to the mouth results. Yet the advertisements still give the clear impression that the right way to treat messy gums, halitosis, and mouth discomfort is to use whatever toothpaste or mouthwash is being touted. The American who relies on the advertising industry for his oral-hygiene information is likely to pay dearly for this misplaced faith.

One may wonder how companies and advertising agencies can get away with fraudulent advertising. Are there no laws to protect the consumer against misrepresentation and fraud? Such laws do exist, but the advertising-copy writers circumvent laws on misrepresentation by never saying anything *explicit* about their products; they are content to misrepresent by suggestion. The advertisement never actually states that XYZ Mouthwash will cure halitosis; instead it says, "XYZ keeps breath fresh for hours." Of course the word *fresh* has no precise meaning. The little lie in *fresh* is reinforced and greatly magnified by the dramatization of the girl's romantic success. The *implication* of her engagement is that her "bad breath" was actually corrected. Under our present laws such a vague but emotionally appealing suggestion cannot be legally pinned down as misrepresentation, though that is what it is.

Occasionally the copy writers do overstep the boundaries of the law by making direct claims that are patently false. The government then prosecutes. Litigation takes years, and even after the government's case is won it turns out that the penalties prescribed by law are no more than a slap on the wrist—perhaps a fine of a few thousand dollars, that must be measured against an advertising budget in the millions, and millions more of profits generated by the fraudulent advertisements. The company is ordered not to repeat the offending advertising, but by now it has launched a new advertising campaign, complete with new lies. Meanwhile the understaffed government agency struggles to prepare a case against some other fraudulent advertiser. Such prosecutions get very little publicity from the advertiser-supported press; you may find such a story occasionally if you search the back pages of the *New York Times* with a reading glass. *Consumer Reports* supplies more regular coverage.

There is much more to be said about advertising, but this should be enough to convince the reader that advertising copy and commercials are not a reliable source of information on oral hygiene—if they are a reliable source of information about anything at all.

12

The Care of
Children's Teeth

The last two decades have seen an increasing emphasis
on dental care for children. In part, the trend very
likely reflects a generally high level of prosperity. But
it is not only the affluent who are concerned for their
children's teeth; I know many parents who, for want
of money, have neglected their own health for years
but still seek the best dental care for their children.
Yet despite the increased interest in dentistry for
children, this field is still the subject of widespread
public ignorance and misinformation.

Many people still believe, for example, that children's
teeth need not be cared for, because they will be lost
anyway. This false and dangerous notion has, as we
shall see, led to major defects of health, appearance,
and personality in a great many people whose entire
lives might have been drastically altered for the better
if they had had the advantage of dental care in their

134

childhood. Other popular beliefs are that baby teeth are easier for the dentist to work on, since he is not required to do such a good job on these "unimportant" teeth, soon to be lost anyway, and that work on baby teeth takes less time and should cost less than work on adult teeth. All of these notions are, as we shall see, completely false.

Everyone knows that there are "baby teeth" and "permanent teeth." The "baby" or "milk" teeth are more scientifically known as the primary or deciduous dentition; the permanent teeth are the secondary or succedaneous dentition. Deciduous teeth differ greatly from the permanent dentition; they are smaller and lighter in color than their successors. Indeed, the first appearance of the permanent front teeth proves disconcerting to many a parent. The new front teeth are three times as large as the tiny deciduous incisors they replace. In addition, the permanent teeth are considerably darker than the adjoining baby teeth; this healthy, accentuated yellowness of the new teeth, coupled with their large size, produces an appearance considerably different from that of the small, even, bluish-white, deciduous incisors they have replaced. Though the new teeth are perfectly normal in both color and size, they may at first appear grotesque to the mother grown accustomed to seeing her child with only tiny, very white, baby-incisors.

The manufacture of a tooth begins long before it erupts, or comes up, through the gum, and continues long after its eruption; this goes for both primary and secondary teeth. The formation of the primary teeth begins as early as the seventh week of pregnancy, although the first teeth to erupt will not make their appearance until about six months after birth. The chronological development of a tooth can be summed up as follows: Tooth-bud formation, beginning of crown formation, completion of crown, beginning of root formation, eruption of tooth, completion of root. Notice especially that it is an incomplete tooth which erupts, the root not being completed for some time afterwards.

A summary of the average schedule of development and eruption of all the baby and permanent teeth is given at the end of this chapter. Bear in mind that this timetable is only the average; the timing may vary quite a bit among healthy children, though the order of eruption is usually the same for all children. Do not be alarmed if your son has no permanent front teeth at age seven while the neighbor's son already has his front teeth by his sixth birthday. But it may be cause for some concern if the development of a child's teeth varies extremely from the average dates suggested in the timetable. In any case, routine check-ups will surely disclose any need for corrective treatment.

The mechanism by which the deciduous teeth are replaced by the permanent dentition is one of the most striking examples of nature's ingenuity. As the permanent tooth develops, it moves through the jaw toward the gums. When it begins to encroach on the area occupied by the root of the deciduous tooth its presence causes a progressive resorption of the root of the deciduous tooth. As the crown of the new tooth continues on its path toward eruption, the baby-tooth root becomes more and more resorbed until, just when the permanent tooth is ready to erupt, the baby-tooth root has virtually disappeared and the baby tooth, having nothing left to hold it in place, drops out. After that the new tooth usually appears very promptly. This mechanism is such that the baby tooth is maintained in the mouth for the longest possible time, even as the permanent tooth is making its progress mouthward. Thus the baby tooth is enabled, up to the last moment, to fulfill its necessary functions in the mouth.

This is very important to the formation of a healthy adult dentition.

In addition to the obvious function of chewing food, the baby teeth also function to guide the development of the jaws and to maintain sufficient space for the eruption of the permanent teeth. A baby tooth that is prematurely lost can no longer serve its function as a space maintainer; some of the remaining teeth may crowd into the gap, and when the time comes for the eruption of the permanent tooth there may be insufficient room for it. The consequences may be quite serious. The tooth may be prevented from erupting at all, and become an *impacted* tooth. If the tooth does erupt, it may erupt in the wrong location, there being insufficient room for eruption at the proper spot. Alternatively, the tooth may force its way into the dental arch, causing crowding and a possible distortion of the whole arch formation. One of the commonest causes of the need for orthodontic treatment, or braces, is the premature loss of deciduous teeth, and the resulting distortions in the arch form and bite.

In addition it must be emphasized that poorly positioned teeth often cause irregularities in jaw formation, and that such irregularities may in turn cause distortions in the profile. The effect upon the individual's personal appearance is then profound. There is little doubt that personal appearance, particularly facial appearance, exerts an enormous influence upon the individual's general success, happiness, and total personality development. It is not far-fetched to say, therefore, that the premature loss of just one baby molar can have the most depressing effect on the course of an entire life. This fact alone should resolve any doubts about the need to care for a child's teeth.

Much of the complexity of the pattern of eruption and development of the permanent teeth can be understood in terms of the development of the first permanent molars, or six-year molars. These are ordinarily the first permanent teeth to make their appearance; they do not replace any of the deciduous teeth, but erupt just behind the last of the baby teeth, the second deciduous molars, while all the deciduous teeth are still in position. The forces of eruption and occlusion tend to drive the new molar teeth anteriorly, to the front part of the mouth, but the deciduous teeth block this anterior migration. The six-year molars are therefore stabilized in position by the presence of the baby teeth. Later on, when it becomes time for the eruption of the permanent premolar teeth that will succeed the baby molar teeth, there will be sufficient room for the new premolars because the baby teeth will have done their job of preventing the six-year molars from moving forward into the territory of the premolars. Should one of the deciduous molars be lost prematurely, then the adjacent six-year molar is likely to migrate anteriorly: When it comes time for the eruption of the premolars, the space originally set aside by nature for the premolars will have been usurped by the migrating first permanent molars. As a result the premolars may become impacted or, if they do succeed in erupting, they may have rotated and be improperly placed. Such a situation will require orthodontic correction at a later date.

There are four first permanent molars, one for each quadrant of the dentition. These teeth are considered by orthodontists to be one of the major keys to occlusion, and dentists can often predict future orthodontic problems by observing the first molars. If the upper and lower six-year molars erupt and develop in normal relationship to each other, then the arch form and bite are likely to be within normal range. If the upper and lower first molars on either side are not in

correct relationship to each other, corrective ortho-
dontics will probably be necessary.

The reason the six-year molars can be used diag-
nostically in this way, at an early age, is that they are
so important to the development of the rest of the
permanent teeth. It is assumed that if these keys to
occlusion are in their proper places, they will do their
job of helping to guide the rest of the permanent dentition into its proper place. The six-year molars themselves serve as space maintainers for the second, or
twelve-year molars. After the loss of the deciduous
molars, between the ages of nine and eleven, there is
a time lapse until the permanent premolars can fully
assume their correct places in the dental arch. During
this time the first molars migrate anteriorly somewhat,
there being no longer any deciduous molars to maintain
the space. But before long the permanent premolars
will have erupted enough to block the further forward
migration of the six-year molars. The reason there is
enough room for this slight anterior migration is that
the baby molar teeth are slightly wider than the permanent premolar teeth which are to replace them. Nature
thinks of everything!

From the standpoint of the development of the final
form of the dentition and the jaws, the first permanent
molars are by far the most important teeth in the
mouth. Yet, as I have seen in the mouths of young
children, these critical teeth are sometimes extracted.
It must take a particularly heartless dentist to remove
such a tooth without making every effort to save it,
since the removal of a child's six-year molar almost
guarantees the poor youngster a very complex orthodontic job or a lifetime of bite disorders, if not both.
The easy extraction policy of so many dentists is particularly reprehensible when it leads to the removal of a
young child's first permanent molar.

The mechanisms involved in the normal pattern of eruption and development are so complex and delicate that it is amazing that things so rarely go wrong. Of those that do, many can be classified as birth defects. Occasionally a permanent tooth is congenitally missing, because the embryonic tooth bud either did not form or was somehow damaged before it was fully developed. This can be a serious problem. The usual treatment is to use a temporary appliance to maintain the space where the missing tooth should be; later, after the eruption of the rest of the teeth and the complete development of the jaws, a fixed bridge can be constructed to replace the tooth. An orthodontic solution can often be found when the same teeth are missing on both sides of the mouth. Another type of congenital defect is an extra tooth, or supernumerary tooth, which may develop in the jaws alongside the normal tooth buds. Sometimes supernumerary teeth are harmless, but they are harmful whenever they interfere with the development, eruption, and placement of the normal teeth. Extra teeth can completely block the eruption of certain teeth, and thus they can cause impactions and serious deformations of the jaws and the dental arch. Usually the best treatment for an offending supernumerary tooth is its removal by surgery. Sometimes this can be a major operation, with important consequences for the future dentition and personal appearance of the individual.

Occasionally some interference with the growth pattern of a tooth produces a congenital malformation. A deformed tooth that proves unsightly or nonfunctional should be treated. Among possible treatments are crown or jacket restorations. But if the tooth is too weak it may have to be extracted. After that the empty space should be maintained until the com-

pletion of final treatment, whether through orthodontia or fixed bridgework.

Trauma is a very common cause of trouble to the
developing teeth. Children are continually falling, getting hit, and getting into all kinds of accidents. Often
these incidents of child violence lead to traumatic
injury to the teeth. A front, baby tooth may be knocked
out some years before it was scheduled to be replaced.
Treatment is rarely necessary in such cases, since the
front teeth do not have the critical space-maintenance
functions of the deciduous molars. While the dentist
should check by means of X-rays for any surgical or
traumatic damage to the permanent tooth buds, it is
very rare that such an injury causes damage to the
developing permanent teeth.

Often a baby front tooth is knocked loose, then
tightens again, and, some time later, turns very dark.
This is because the tooth was displaced in its socket
in the jaw, and the tiny capillaries and nervelets which
supply the pulp of the tooth were torn. Thus the tooth
lost its blood supply, its source of nourishment for the
pulp, which now degenerates and discolors the tooth.
As a rule, no treatment is necessary in such cases, since
by the time the dying pulp becomes gangrenous, so that
it might give trouble, it is time for the tooth to be
replaced anyway; baby front teeth are usually lost by
age seven. Although injuries of this type are common
and not often serious, it is not easy for a parent to be
casual about them. The child usually comes home in
pain, screaming. Typically the lip is greatly swollen
and bloodied, sticking straight out; the gum is swollen,
purplish-blue, and oozing blood; and the tooth is quite
loose. The child, sensing the parents' anxiety, howls
all the more hysterically. Yet, as a rule, the pain soon
goes away, the swelling goes down in a day or two,

and the child forgets about the wound. But as a pre-caution he should nevertheless be checked promptly for serious injury.

By far the most common cause of serious trouble to the developing dentition of a child is the premature loss of a deciduous molar, and this factor is of course controllable. If such a tooth should be lost, however, prompt construction of a space-maintaining appliance is usually advisable. But the best way to avoid possibly grave consequences for the child's future health and personal appearance is, by properly caring for his teeth, to see that they are not prematurely lost. And yet a great many laymen, and even some *dentists,* still be-lieve that baby teeth are unimportant, and need not be cared for. After all, these people reason, those teeth will be falling out soon enough anyway. This absurd attitude has been encouraged by some dentists who don't want to make the effort or take the time to work on children's teeth. They should at least be sufficiently responsible and compassionate to send the child to an-other dentist who is willing to work on children. Neglect of a child's teeth by his parents is bad enough, but planned neglect by the child's *dentist* is unspeakable. Suffice it to say that a child's teeth deserve as careful care as do the teeth of an adult, and that failure to provide good care can have irreparable consequences. To that often-asked question, must we bother with children's teeth, there is only one answer, a loud, un-equivocal Yes!

The dental training of children should start early. Tooth-brushing should start as soon as the child has a significant number of teeth to be brushed. At this stage, of course, the child lacks the dexterity to do a proper job, and the parent should complete the brushing session started by the child. The child's first visit to the dentist should take place at about age two.

Just as there are many dentists who do not treat children, so there are others who have limited their practice to pedodontia, or children's dentistry, which has been growing as a dental specialty. Fear is a widespread cause of dental neglect. If this fear can be corrected when the child is young, then the crippling effects of dental neglect caused by fear will never affect the adult. The pedodontist usually orients his facilities and the whole of his office routine to the psychological needs of the child. Waiting rooms are supplied with children's books, games, and dental-education materials. A few offices even have toy trains, and I have heard of some with live pets. A capable pedodontist uses special techniques to relieve a child's anxieties, and he can transform a terrified child into a good, cooperative patient who is no longer afraid of dental treatment. The pedodontist's aim is just this, and his fee, which may seem high, is justified by this achievement alone, regardless of the actual dental work he accomplishes.

The psychological and other techniques employed by the pedodontist are exactly the same as those used by any dentist who treats children properly. The child coming to a new dentist for the first time is often a bagful of anxieties. His knowledge of dentistry has been obtained from his little friends; his mind teems with fearful thoughts of the drill, the needle, and the pain he expects the dentist to inflict on him. His parents, particularly if their dental experience has been of the Poorwork variety, have reinforced the child's fears with their own anxieties, either deliberately or inadvertently. Children are alert and perceptive, and they pick up attitudes from the parents without the parents ever suspecting. If the child has had a previous experience with Dr. Poorwork's speed-up dentistry, then the job of the pedodontist will be that much harder now that

Poorwork has confirmed and cemented all the child's fears. It is this little bundle of anxieties which now confronts the dentist; it will be his job to get this horrified child to open his mouth and submit to procedures which may not be actually painful, but which will surely be uncomfortable and inconvenient. If he is to succeed, the dentist must call on his experience and training in child psychology and the techniques for handling the child. These days all dentists have had such training, but success often requires a great deal of time and patience. The pedodontist is willing to spend the time, and he expects to be paid for it.

The principles and techniques of child psychology are basic to the expertise of all dentists who treat children. By discussing these principles and techniques here I hope to help parents to gain a keener understanding of what the pedodontist, or any dentist who treats children, is trying to do, and of some of the problems he faces.

Children are smart, they are alert, and they are perceptive. They have superb memories, and *they cannot be fooled.* They expect candid and honest behavior from the dentist, and their acute memories can be embarrassing. If, for example, a child is promised something for the next visit, or the dentist mentions that he will be doing a certain procedure next time, the child will remember, and if the dentist forgets his promise or omits the procedure that he mentioned, there will be trouble. Because he knows children, the good dentist never attempts to deceive a child, who would see through a deception in any case. Dr. Poorwork, hiding an injection syringe or a drill or a forceps behind his back, sneaking up on the child patient, is never able to do proper work; the child does not trust him enough to let him. What is worse, the child who has experienced such deception may never be amenable to dental care, unless he is very carefully handled by his next dentist.

Children are not moral theoreticians. Although they demand unrelenting honesty and candor from the dentist, they continually challenge him with deceptions of their own. The dentist must be alert enough to detect each childish deception, and he must inform the child in a firm manner that he, the dentist, is not being fooled. The child will respect consistency and firmness; these qualities are offshoots of honesty. But it may be troublesome for the dentist to maintain consistency. For example, any change in procedure from one visit to another may make the child suspect that something is being put over on him. Most dentists try to standardize their operative procedures as much as possible, lest the child, noticing a change in methods, become suspicious. I have heard children complain because, between visits, I had switched to a germicide of a slightly different color without telling them; they thought I was doing something essentially different.

The dentist can confidently expect to treat even the difficult child successfully, because he knows that, using modern techniques, including local anesthesia, the dental work will not hurt. True enough, the work may prove to be uncomfortable and inconvenient, but there will not be such pain that the child will be really distressed *once the work is under way.* That is the catch. The difficult child expects to be hurt, and the dentist's job is to get him to allow the dental work to begin. Once it has begun, the child learns that it actually does not hurt and he develops confidence that further work will not hurt either, if the dentist says it won't. Then the battle is won.

But first the dentist must induce the child to allow some work to be done. To make the task easier all around, the dentist begins with an easy goal, such as counting the teeth. He announces his plan very clearly. "Today I am going to count your teeth," he says to the child. After that, come what may, the dentist *must* at least count the child's teeth on this visit. This may not be easy. Some children throw a tantrum at the sight of the chair, or even at the sight of the dentist's uniform. Nevertheless, the dentist must persist, using *whatever means is necessary,* except dishonesty or deception, to accomplish the counting of the teeth. In extreme cases he may have to resort to force, but whatever means is necessary, the child *must* sit in that chair and have his teeth counted.

If the child is difficult, the counting of the teeth is enough work for the first visit. It is no small accomplishment, however. Once the teeth have been counted, the child will have learned that what the dentist says goes, and that if the dentist says that teeth are going to counted, then *those teeth will be counted.* The child has also learned that what transpired was not painful, that the dentist was completely honest and made no attempt to deceive him, and that there were no unpleasant surprises; everything that happened was told to him beforehand. This first visit can be crucial to the success of later treatment, and it can be most demanding upon the dentist's time, skill, and emotional resources. The specialist in pedodontia may charge twenty-five dollars and up for such a visit, just to count the teeth, and it is well worth it.

This first visit often emerges as a contest between child and practitioner. The child feels more secure if he loses. If he wins, he will never permit the dentist to work on him in peace. Fortunately, the dentist has many advantages. He is much bigger and stronger than the child and can manipulate the child physically if need be; he is also, we hope, smarter than the child, and can see through all the child's deceptions. At each attempt to deceive him, the dentist must make the child understand clearly that he is not being fooled.

In this struggle, both sides will look to the parents for support. The child may be accustomed to manipulating the parents at will, and so the dentist must make absolutely certain of the parents' full cooperation beforehand. The dentist should be friendly, kind, and understanding, and he must smile easily, but he must tolerate no nonsense. He should become extremely stern, if necessary, but he should always be ready to be friendly again as the child becomes more compliant. The dentist must not react emotionally; children are impressed by a stern, forceful manner, but are contemptuous of rage. He must also be careful what he says. Words with emotional content, such as *hurt* and *pain,* should never be used with a new patient, and should be avoided even with an experienced patient. Perhaps the greatest demand put upon the discipline, intelligence, and experience of the dentist is the necessity to maintain a perfect consistency in both words and action.

Typically, much of the child's fear of the dentist has been transmitted from the parents. The cooperative parent, especially one who is properly instructed, can nevertheless be enormously helpful. The dentist should therefore have a private talk with one or both of the parents before the first visit, to explain just what he plans to do. If the parent withholds full approval of the practitioner's methods, the dentist should decline to treat the child.

The parent should be instructed to watch, and to hold the child's hand if the child wishes, but to say *nothing.* Since the parent is untrained, and is likely to say just the wrong thing, any words about the treatment must come from the dentist. The parent who looks sympathetically at the child and says, "Don't cry, he won't hurt you," may have sabotaged a half-hour of careful psychological preparatory work by the dentist. The parent who says, "Sit still for one minute, then I'll buy you an ice cream," or, "It will be all over in one minute," or, "Wait until your father hears about this," or, "We're going right home if you don't behave," is probably destroying the whole purpose of the visit. When the child looks appealingly at the parent for help, the parent must make it understood that the dentist is the boss, and that the parent is merely an onlooker. Unfortunately many parents find it impossible to remain aloof when their child is in tears or even hysterical, and is being sternly handled by the dentist. On occasion, I have had to refuse treatment to children after the parents had proved themselves unable to cooperate.

The parent, preferably the mother, should be in the room; her presence reassures the child that he is not in completely hostile country. A parent's steadfast support of the dentist gives him further authority, and he often finds that using that authority by threatening to send the parent from the room helps establish initial control of the child. After several minutes of listening to the child cry, the dentist may say, "Stop crying or I send Mother out of the room." The child may doubt that the dentist possesses such formidable authority, and may test the dentist by crying the louder. "All right, Mother, you have to leave the room," says the dentist, and Mother, previously briefed, does so. "Mother can return when you stop crying," the child is told. After a few more strong wails the child realizes that the dentist is not kidding, and he stops crying. "Come on back, Mother," orders the dentist, and sure enough, Mother reappears.

This is likely to impress the child greatly, though he usually tries crying again. Again the dentist counters with the threat to remove Mother if he does not stop. If he still cries, Mother is promptly sent out again, to return as soon as the crying stops. By this time the child usually gets the idea. I do not wish to appear heartless in the treatment of this poor, crying child, so please remember that he is crying without having had any work done upon him. Though he is in the dental chair, he still has not even opened his mouth so that his teeth could be counted. He is crying out of fear and frustration at not having his own way. He will stop crying only when he realizes that this dentist cannot be wheedled and fooled the way his mother can, that his fear is unfounded, and that he can feel secure in the authority and reliability of the dentist, this powerful man who can banish his mother at will and yet faithfully keeps his promise to bring her back as soon as his conditions are met.

The first visit is the one most likely to produce commotion and hysterics; only rarely does a second or third of these orientation sessions prove necessary. After the child develops the desired understanding with the dentist, there will rarely be any more noise or hysterics. Once the child learns he will not be fooled or hurt, he will sit in the dental chair without complaining, open his mouth wide, and quietly put up with the most complex dental procedures. He even leaves with a smile on his face, and he will never again in his lifetime have an unreasonable terror of the dentist. These results are so obviously desirable that the parent who understands should readily agree to whatever measures are necessary at the first visit, even to the extent of quietly accepting some hysterics and even, possibly, some roughhouse.

At this point I had better interject that *the previous paragraphs deal only with treating the difficult child, who is the one most likely to be seen by a specialist.*

With the average child who is not already transfixed with fear of the dentist, the approach will be the same, but hysterics and commotion will not be the order of the day. In most cases the orientation visit goes smoothly; if the counting of the teeth is uneventful, as it usually is, the dentist can proceed directly with an X-ray examination. On the same first visit he can also introduce the child to some of his instruments, such as the mouth mirror and the explorer, or "pointer," and demonstrate their use first on models, and then in the mouth. But of course the dentist does *nothing* without thoroughly explaining and demonstrating it to the child first. With the typical child all this usually proceeds smoothly.

Only in the case of a badly frightened, difficult child will major problems be encountered. Ultimately, with great patience on the part of both dentist and parents, the difficult child's orientation will have been completed and his confidence gained. Only then can restorative dental procedures begin. In nearly every case in my recollection, X-rays and cleaning were accomplished by the end of the second visit, while restorative work usually started by the third visit, if not by the second.

The treatment of children's teeth is essentially the same as for adult teeth, though there are some differences. Baby teeth are somewhat different structurally from adult teeth. They are smaller, and there is less thickness of hard tissue, enamel and dentin, to protect the pulp. There is therefore less room for the dentist to drill before he exposes the pulp. The preparations of the teeth are modified somewhat because of these differences. The other important consideration is that within a short time the baby teeth will fall out and be replaced by the permanent teeth. It would not make sense to make a major restoration for a tooth that will come out naturally in a few month's time, nor is it sensible to fill a very small cavity on a tooth soon to be lost. Yet a decaying baby tooth must be treated if it is scheduled to stay in the mouth for any length of time; it should not be permitted to abscess and thus be lost prematurely. The dentist is able to judge, from X-rays and the clinical appearance of the tooth, if the tooth should be treated or if it is very nearly ready to come out and be replaced.

Aside from the considerations mentioned above, the treatment of baby teeth and permanent teeth is about the same. It is as difficult, if not more so, to fill a deciduous tooth as it is to fill an analogous cavity in a permanent tooth. For identical dental work, aside from orientation and problems with difficult children, a general dentist's fees for children's dentistry should be comparable to fees for adult dentistry.

Time, as we have seen elsewhere in these pages, is the indispensable key to success in all phases of dentistry, and children's dentistry is no exception. Dr. Poorwork, who is unwilling to spend time on any phase of dentistry, either refuses entirely to work on children's teeth, or else he does the most perfunctory sort of job, often as he holds the child down physically, since his appointment book is too crowded for him to take the time for better methods. Later on, when the job has failed and the pulp has become infected, Poorwork can always collect another fee for extracting the tooth.

Not all dentists who refuse to work on children's teeth are Poorworks. In fact, many excellent dentists consider themselves temperamentally unsuited to the emotional demands of children's dentistry. They are right to refer children to a pedodontist. The alternative would be to make a weak attempt to treat children, with potentially bad results both to the patients and to the practitioner.

But Dr. Poorwork often neglects a child's mouth while pretending to treat it, or perhaps while shrugging the problem off as "just a little difficulty with the temporary baby teeth," because he is unwilling to spend the needed time with the child. He compounds his own failure to treat the child by not referring him to a pedodontist; he prefers, instead, to extract those teeth that become most seriously decayed. Poorwork has what he considers his own good and sufficient reasons for not referring the child to a children's dentist. One reason is that he doesn't want the parents to witness the painstaking methods of the pedodontist, or to learn from him that filling a tooth takes time. Poorwork also fears that the parent who is accustomed to his "reasonable" fees will object strongly to the specialist's fees, which are high even in comparison to those of a good general dentist. "What kind of a crook did you send me to?" is a kind of question Poorwork does not want to hear from his patients. The same sort of objection is unlikely to be raised by patients of the good dentist, who are better informed about dental problems and therefore know that money spent now can avert serious health problems and much larger expenditures in the future.

Should "problem children" be referred to men who specialize in dentistry under general anesthesia? Dentistry performed under such conditions certainly has its uses in the case of genuinely unmanageable patients, including some cerebral palsy victims, psychotics, and others. A high percentage of the patients of general-anesthesia dentists are adults who are absolutely terrified of the dentist, and who don't want to know what is going on. But general anesthesia is not an experience we want a child to associate with dentistry. To be unconscious during dental work is not to understand what is going on, and not to understand, in this case, is to be afraid. Perhaps many of the terrified adults who go to general-anesthesia dentists would never have found themselves in such an unhappy predicament if they had received more considerate dental treatment when they were children.

Working with general anesthesia presents many difficulties. Dentists often want the patient to cooperate actively, as by holding a cotton roll, tilting his head, moving his jaw, opening wider, and so on. But unconscious patients are unable to cooperate; their mouths must be propped open, and the depth of the anesthesia must be checked almost continuously. And it is understandable that when there is a great deal of work to be done, the dentist who uses full anesthesia will try to treat as many teeth as possible in each session, in order to hold the number of sessions to a minimum. Such conditions are not conducive to the best dentistry; judging from what I have seen, the man who can produce adequate dental work under them is rare indeed. It is unfortunate, then, that some dentists refer their so-called unmanageable child patients to dentists who use general anesthesia. But really unmanageable children are less common than some distracted parents and hurried dentists may think. In my first thirteen years of practice I have encountered only one child whom I would call genuinely unmanageable. There have also been a handful of others whom I have refused to treat because of lack of parental cooperation. My experience is similar to that of many dentists and pedodontists I know.

When Dr. Poorwork refers a child to anyone, it is often to a man specializing in general anesthesia rather than to a pedodontist. Dr. Poorwork does not want his patients to see what good dentistry is like and what it can accomplish, as demonstrated by a skillful and patient pedodontist. On the other hand, the results achieved by the general-anesthesia dentist are often similar to those Poorwork himself gets: bad! With him, Poorwork runs no risk of unfavorable comparison.

Timetable of the Development and Eruption of the Teeth

The timetable set forth below merely represents the average behavior of the teeth of all children. It is not necessarily significant if an individual child's teeth do not erupt strictly in accordance with the schedule.

The formation of the embryonic tooth buds of the primary teeth begins as early as the seventh week of pregnancy; by the fourth month of pregnancy the hard structures of these teeth have begun to form. At birth none of the primary teeth have their complete crowns, but within two months the central incisors will have completed crown formation, and before one year all of the baby teeth will have completely formed crowns, though most will still be beneath the gums. The eruption of the first teeth starts at about six months, and by the age of two all the baby teeth have made their appearance. The development of the roots continues after eruption; the roots of all the primary dentition are not completed until sometime between the third and fourth year of age.

Some of the permanent teeth have their embryonic beginnings before birth, and at birth the first permanent molars have already begun to calcify. These first molars make their appearance at the age of six years, usually while all the deciduous teeth are still in position. After the eruption of the six-year molars the baby teeth begin to loosen and be lost, each being replaced in turn by an erupting permanent tooth. The deciduous centrals and laterals are lost between the ages of six and nine, the deciduous molars between nine and eleven. By about age twelve all of the deciduous teeth have been replaced by permanent teeth, and the permanent second molars, or the twelve-year molars, are erupting. The pattern of eruption is completed somewhere between the ages of fifteen and twenty-five with the uncertain appearance of the third molars, or wisdom teeth.

13

A Smattering of Oral Medicine

Many drugs and chemicals are employed in the dentist's office, and there are other medicines that people use in the hope of obtaining relief from various types of dental discomfort. Although many of these remedies are virtually useless, there are some dental medicines of special interest. Several of these are briefly discussed here, together with the dental condition associated with the remedy.

Toothache and Postoperative Pain

"My tooth is hurting. What can I take for it?" This is a question often asked me at parties, on the beach, and over the telephone. Unfortunately there is no really good answer. The only effective way to deal with dental pain is to correct whatever causes it, and this cannot be done over the phone or away from the dentist's office, and it certainly cannot be done with a drug. Yet there are many preparations designed to ease dental pain; some of these may be of some help until the patient can get to the dentist.

The "poultice," an old-fashioned but still-used toothache remedy, generally available in drug stores, consists of a small sack of drugs to be laid on the gum next to the tooth that aches. The poultice is a counterirritant; its contents irritate the surrounding gum and jawbone, producing an additional center of pain, so that the responses of the body are no longer concentrated entirely on the toothache. Oddly enough, this type of medication occasionally is somewhat effective, though usually not for severe toothaches. The classical example of a counterirritant is the mustard plaster, which is supposed to relieve the deep discomfort of a chest cold by irritating the superficial tissues. Whether the poultice works or not, the aim of the person with a toothache should be to see a dentist as soon as he can do so.

Aspirin is still the most commonly used and least harmful pain-killing drug. It is also amazingly effective; in fact aspirin is the strongest pain-killer you can buy without a prescription. All pain-killing proprietary nonprescription drugs that are in any way effective contain aspirin, and aspirin is the only really effective ingredient in any of them. Aspirin is usually strong enough to relieve a minor toothache or the postoperative pain of dental work, but one should not expect this drug to relieve an acute toothache or severe postoperative dental pain. (The latter is rare.) A dentist who anticipates a severely painful reaction to his work prescribes a stronger pain-killer, usually a narcotic preparation.

A word of caution: Aspirin is to be taken internally only. Some people believe that aspirin relieves toothache pain if the tablets are placed in the fold of the cheek next to the tooth. This is a serious mistake; when aspirin is applied externally it can cause severe tissue burns.

Eugenol, the active principle of oil of cloves, which is responsible for the charactistic smell of the dental office, is one of the few really useful dental medications. It is an effective sedative for the pulp of the tooth and one of the few medications that can calm down a hyperemic, or sensitive, tooth. Dentists use this drug as a base for most temporary filling materials, relying on its sedative properties to diminish the pain of a sensitive tooth. It is often used in intermediate fillings during procedures, such as pulp-capping, which might be likely to cause postoperative pain. Eugenol is also the active ingredient in the so-called toothache drops sold at drug stores.

Despite the many legitimate uses of eugenol, it is also a much-abused medication, particularly in Poorwork-style dentistry. The sedative effect of eugenol is often used by the Poorworks to control pain in lieu of careful removal of all decay. One of the most typical Poorwork procedures is a hasty and perfunctory drilling that removes some of the decay from a deep cavity, and the placing of a temporary filling containing eugenol to control pain. At a subsequent visit the tooth receives a so-called permanent filling. Such treatment of deep cavities is still most popular with the Poorworks, because it takes so little time relative to what is needed to excavate *all* the decay. The career of teeth treated in this way often terminates in extraction.

Sensitivity to Temperature

One of the most frustrating puzzles is that of apparently healthy teeth which occasionally demonstrate a sharp sensitivity to temperature change, usually toward cold, and perhaps to certain foods, usually sweets. The sensitive teeth are usually those which have large restorations, but teeth with no dental work also have shown these symptoms. Many explanations have been advanced for such sensitivity, and its treatment is often quite frustrating to dentist and patient.

Silver nitrate is one of the chemicals commonly employed to reduce this sensitivity. The dentist applies the silver nitrate, a powerful caustic agent, to the sensitive part of the tooth, almost always at the gum line, in an attempt to cauterize the sensitive surface and thereby reduce the pain. This procedure often shows initial success, though the sensitivity often returns. It is claimed that certain toothpastes improve sensitive teeth, but these preparations are less successful than silver nitrate. Other chemicals have been used, all with little success. Dentistry still awaits an effective treatment for occasionally sensitive, otherwise healthy teeth.

Denture Complaints

There are a number of proprietary preparations ("brand-name") designed to relieve discomfort caused by dentures. The ointments and liquids to be put on denture sores contain a local anesthetic that will indeed relieve the pain. But as a rule such pain is caused by a bad fit in some area of the denture; unless this situation is corrected, the pain will always return as soon as the anesthetic wears off. Denture sores should be taken to the dentist, who generally has little difficulty in correcting whatever it is that causes them. Anesthetic preparations should be used only under his supervision. People who use pain-killing ointments, except on the dentist's advice, may perpetuate an irritation of the gums, with serious, even lethal consequences.

Advertised denture-cleaning pastes, denture adhesives, and soak-overnight cleaners are discussed in the chapter on Oral Hygiene. Here it should be enough to say that, in general, none of these should be used, except perhaps for the *occasional* use of a cleaning paste. The adhesives are capable of causing damage to the tissues, and incautious use of a cleaning paste may damage the denture. Relining materials, discussed in the chapter on Full Dentures, should *never* be applied by anybody but a dentist; improper relining can have the most serious consequences.

Canker Sores and Cold Sores

The canker sore, or apthous ulcer, is one of the best-known and most persistently annoying dental lesions. It is small and whitish, and may occur on the gums or cheeks, or under the tongue. It appears singly and in clusters. The sore is usually quite painful, and is especially sensitive to the touch and to hot or spicy foods, but fortunately it runs its course in about a week to ten days. No good treatment for it is known; cortisone preparations have been tried recently, with occasional success, and attempts are being made to develop a vaccine. Some people are especially prone to canker sores, and there may be a connection between canker attacks and emotional stress, though there is still no definite information on the causes of this puzzling disorder.

Fever blisters, also known as cold sores, may be related to the canker sore, and may also be connected in some way to the common cold or to unknown irritants. Cold sores resemble canker sores in that there is no really effective treatment for them. They just have to run their course.

Trouble with Wisdom Teeth

Pericoronitis (peri = around, corona = crown, itis = inflammation) is a condition known to most teenagers who are cutting their wisdom teeth. It is a painful inflammation, usually infectious, which develops around the crown of an erupting wisdom tooth. Most wisdom teeth are at least partially impacted, which is to say that the teeth are "stuck" in the jaw because there is not enough room for them to erupt fully. In such cases, with the tooth half in and half out, a flap of gum tissue is produced. This flap is a marvelous food trap and source of infection. Pericoronal infections can become quite serious; for this reason they should be treated promptly by the dentist. Signs of pericoronitis include pain and swelling in the area of the wisdom tooth, and difficulty in opening the mouth, especially in the morning. Hot salt water rinses will help clean the area and possibly help draw out the infection. The ultimate treatment for pericoronitis is usually the removal of the impacted wisdom tooth; as a temporary treatment, the dentist may wish to establish drainage for the infection and to cleanse the area.

Tongue Troubles

"Geographic tongue" is a condition in which patches migrate from one area of the tongue to another. Not much is known about this condition, which is fairly common and apparently harmless. *"Black, hairy tongue"* is an unappealing though perfectly descriptive term given to a tongue condition often caused by routine use of a peroxide or perborate type of mouthwash. The picturesque though unesthetic condition usually disappears promptly after the mouthwash is discontinued.

The tongue often has some sort of coating on it. (If you stand in front of a mirror and stick your tongue all the way out, you may be surprised at what you see, especially if you are a smoker.) The doctor of old used his knowledge of tongue coatings in diagnosis; "Stick out your tongue" was usually the first thing he said to a patient. Today's physician, who relies on an array of new drugs and diagnostic tests, has lost the art of interpreting tongue coatings. When is the last time you heard a doctor say, "Stick out your tongue?"

Lumps in the Cheeks

There is a structure in the mouth the discovery of which often panics patients. This is the opening of Stenson's duct, from the parotid, which is one of the salivary glands. Stenson's duct is located on the inside of the cheek, opposite the molar teeth; there is one on each side of the mouth. Some people live half their lives without realizing that they have this little structure on the cheek. When they at last find it, they are conviced they have cancer. If you see such a swelling on your cheek, check to see if there is one just like it on the other side. If there is, it is Stenson's duct you have discovered.

Cancer

The dentist is trained to detect oral cancer; any suspicious or abnormal lesion, swelling, or sore in or around the mouth should be reported to him. Cancers can arise from irritations caused by ill-fitting dentures, and chemical and mechanical irritations caused by smoking can lead to cancer of mouth, lip, or tongue. Dental check-ups should include careful inspection of all the mouth tissues for signs of any untoward lesions.

Antibiotics: Abuses and Some Uses.

History's most spectacular chapter in the treatment of disease has been written in the past twenty-five years by the antibiotics. The handling of these drugs by doctors and dentists has been much less spectacular. In fact, our use of them has been so thoughtless and selfish that we may be destroying their effectiveness and, at the same time, unleashing vicious biological forces. Future generations, far from viewing these times as a glorious chapter in medicine, may come to regard our era as a most dismal chapter, and all because of the stupid overuse of these miracle drugs.

I remember, nearly twenty years ago, listening to a lecture given to a group of students by one of the men who pioneered the antibiotics. He spoke of a world-wide evolution of microbes, which ordinarily would take millions of years, being accomplished in a few decades under the stimulus of the new drugs. He warned us strongly against what might happen if the drugs were used carelessly. He said that new strains of antibiotic-resistant bacteria would develop, and that in time these would render the miracle drugs all but useless, and open the floodgates to uncontrollable disease. Finally, he warned us not to rely on science's ability always to find new drugs to fight the new bacteria.

The prophecy has not yet been fulfilled, but penicillin, the earliest and the most widely used of the drugs, has lost a good bit of its effectiveness, and it is no longer useful against some infectious conditions that, not long ago, were completely controlled by this drug. Many staphylococcal infections no longer respond to penicillin. This is not because penicillin is weaker today than it was twenty-five years ago, but because it has been so overused that the bacteria have evolved resistant forms. The experience with penicillin has caused the medical profession to be somewhat more cautious in the use of the newer drugs, but the antibiotics are still grossly overused.

Two people are suffering from heavy colds. One goes to Dr. A, who tells him to take aspirin, keep warm, and stay home for a few days. The other goes to Dr. P, who gives him a shot of penicillin. After a few days the two colds run their course, and both men are back at work. Dr. P's patient is probably over his cold the least bit sooner, and the antibiotic protects him against possible infectious complications. But though P's patient received the wrong treatment, he probably regards P as the better physician. Dr. A refrained from using antibiotics because he considered complications highly unlikely, because he did not wish to expose his patient to the possibility of an allergic reaction or other side-effect, and because he did not want to contribute to a further weakening of the antibiotics. Dr. P, on the other hand, was trying to develop a reputation as a faster healer and a thoroughly modern doctor. The treatment given by Dr. P, though it is bad practice, is more likely to be appreciated by an uninformed public.

Aside from war and an accidental thermonuclear disaster, scientists consider that the most serious threats to life on our planet are: pollution of the air and water by industrial and chemical wastes; the indiscriminate use of pesticides and chemicals, such as bacteriocidal detergents; and the misuse of chemical agents, particularly the antibiotics, that affect the life processes. With all this in mind, what I now have to say should come as no surprise. It is my belief that antibiotics should be used in dentistry very rarely, if at all. With few exceptions, dental infections can be successfully treated without them. In fact, the nonantibiotic treatments are generally more effective, because, unlike the antibiotics, they remove the cause of infection, and not merely the infection itself, which can always return. As long as the cause remains, the infection is likely to recur.

Antibiotics should be used as a prophylactic measure before surgical procedures on patients with heart trouble. Otherwise their use should be restricted to the treatment of massive infections, or as a treatment of last resort. I doubt if I use antibiotics as much as twice a year in my practice.

The Smells and Tastes of the Dentist's Office

Patients are often curious about the peculiar aromas and flavors that they encounter in the dental office. The medication that is most widely used by dentists is eugenol, which comes from oil of cloves and smells and tastes the way you might expect—like cloves. The odor like that of formaldehyde might come from formocresol or chloroform, both of which are used, often with eugenol, in root canal treatment. Many impression materials are artificially flavored to make their use less unpleasant. Acetone, which is responsible for the characteristic odor of nail-polish removers, is used as a solvent to trim certain types of cavity insulators; acrylic plastics, used in some restorations, have an acetone-like smell. And if you smell something like varnish the next time you visit the dentist, the odor probably comes from a type of cavity insulator.

Transplants and Implants

Much has been heard lately about the controversial procedures of transplants and implants. Transplants are anything but new; indeed, the Romans did tooth transplants two thousand years ago, but they probably had no greater success than is obtained today. Appliance implants, which are metal fixtures inserted into the jawbone to support false teeth, are newer, but in my opinion equally dubious at this stage of development. Appliance implants do offer some promise for the future, once the present difficulties are resolved.

PART 3

SOME MAJOR PROBLEMS AND RESTORATIONS

14

Crowns and Jackets

When the word *crown* is used in its restorative sense it refers to an artificial crown which restores a defective or badly decayed crown of a tooth by covering it. A jacket is an esthetic crown, usually of porcelain or plastic, used mainly to restore front teeth. Crowns and jackets are often called by the unprofessional term *caps*. A national newsweekly recently made me shudder by referring to the "capping service" offered by dentists. This misnomer appeared in an article that was packed with the sort of misinformation that the average person has about dentistry. The article reminded me how difficult it is for the layman to obtain any real information about the teeth and dentistry, and, in fact, it was this magazine piece that finally made me decide to write this book.

The properly made crown is an excellent restoration. Regardless of the extent of the decay, almost any tooth with a periodontally sound root can be salvaged with a crown. Even teeth with their natural crowns decayed right down to the root can often be saved by "post-crown" restorations. Except in the case of periodontally hopeless teeth, the idea that a tooth may be nonre-storable has almost vanished from good, modern dentistry. Nowadays there is almost no such thing as a tooth too badly decayed to be saved.

Crowns are used for many purposes besides restoring otherwise hopeless teeth. Well-made full crowns are the most solid abutments for fixed bridges and fixed perio-dontal splints. In many types of partial dentures, crowns placed on the abutment teeth are used as preci-sion attachments or to facilitate clasping. But in any elaborate fixed-bridgework procedure, splint, or re-habilitation, the restoration can be no better than the individual crowns involved. Crowns and jackets are also used for strictly esthetic purposes. (See chapter on Cosmetic Dentistry.

There are some common fallacies concerning crowns and their purposes. When a man says, "I have just had my teeth capped," his statement often leads to the assumption that he had the "caps" made for the sake of appearance, or because in some mysterious way they strengthen the teeth. When another layman says, "My dentist told me that either I have my teeth capped or I will lose them," you can be fairly sure that the speaker has no clear understanding of his own words or, what is worse, his own oral situation. It is true that many crowns are made just to improve appearance, but most crowns are made to improve, restore and maintain function. A single crown on a single tooth will not strengthen the tooth; but as part of a periodontal splint the multiple attached crowns will pool their strength and lend support to periodontally weak teeth. In this way the teeth will be strengthened, and this may explain the patient's statement that either his teeth must be capped, or he would lose them.

Once a crown is decided upon, the next step is the preparation of the tooth, a procedure which includes the grinding away of a considerable bulk of tooth structure. This bulk reduction was a tiresome job before the advent of the high-speed drills, but is now accomplished much more easily. The details of the work vary in several different specialized types of preparations that can be used to make a tooth ready to receive a crown; each type has its advocates. Whatever kind of preparation is chosen, the dentist must execute it with great care. Through the grinding process, in any case, the tooth is rendered more or less cone-shaped, with slightly tapering walls, so as to receive the crown, which must go on over the tooth. If the prepared tooth were not slightly cone-shaped and tapered, the crown could not be made to fit over it, and an accurate fit could not be achieved. A number of variations in the preparation are directly related to the type of crown to be made. A preparation for a porcelain jacket, for example, requires a ledge to be cut around the part of the preparation ending at the gum. This ledge, called a *shoulder,* is necessary because of the limitations of the particular material. To be strong, porcelain must have a certain minimum thickness; cutting the shoulder in the tooth allows for this minimum thickness. Gold, on the other hand, is still strong even when finished to a knife-edge, so shoulder preparations are not necessary for gold crowns. If a crown is to be veneered for esthetic reasons, a shoulder must first be prepared in the area of the intended veneer to allow for sufficient bulk of the veneering material.

Having completed the grinding of the tooth, the dentist now proceeds with impressions. There are many techniques for making these. Old-fashioned impression compound, a mixture of waxes and resins that has been in use for years, used in a copper impression band delivers excellent results. Although compound is time-consuming and difficult to use, it is still employed by many fine dentists. Satisfactory impression techniques using other materials have recently been developed. These include silicone and rubber-base materials, and hydrocolloid. Needless to say, all methods have their partisans. After the impression of the prepared tooth has been taken, further impressions are taken to register the bite and the jaw relationships as well as the position of the prepared tooth relative to the adjoining teeth. Again, various methods are available. Once all this is completed, the dentist fashions a temporary crown to protect the newly ground-down tooth and to maintain its relative position in the mouth. An appointment is then made for another day, to allow time for the crown to be cast. A method for the laboratory casting of gold is described in the chapter on Decay.

At the next visit the dentist will have the rough-cast crown ready for fitting to the tooth. This fitting visit is crucial. The crown is seated on the prepared tooth and painstakingly checked for contact with adjacent teeth, occlusion, and, most important, marginal fit. The crown should be so finished at the margins that tooth and crown blend; there should be no sticking out of the margin or end of the crown. Sometimes X-rays are necessary to verify marginal fit. The different types of faulty margins can be dangerous in many ways. If the margin is short, it will leave some of the tooth uncovered and unprotected. If the margin is too long, it will impinge on the gums and produce periodontal damage. If the margin stands away from the tooth, it will catch food and retain it against the unprotected part of the root; root decay is likely to result. Such margins also chronically irritate the periodontal tissues and can be expected to accelerate bone loss in the area, much as would a heavy piece of subgingival calculus.

A margin that stands away from the tooth *must* be corrected. Some improper margins can be trimmed on the die; to facilitate such trimming, dies are usually made of metal. If the margin cannot be corrected, the crown must be remade from new impressions. Once the margins are satisfactorily trimmed, and all other necessary adjustments made, the crown is polished and cemented in place. If the crown is to be veneered for the sake of esthetics, the color match is ascertained and the veneering is done before cementation.

Cementation of the finished crown requires care. A crown that is well made will fit exactly, leaving little room between crown and tooth for cement. The cement must therefore be mixed extremely thin, so that it will not interfere with the exact seating of the crown. The cemented crown should have but the thinnest layer of cement between it and the tooth. In fact, the crown that fits well does not rely on the cement to keep it in place. The role of the cement is mainly to provide a seal, and to serve as insulation. A proper seal prevents leakage of oral fluids, food debris, and bacterial exudate under the crown and against the tooth. It should be clear, therefore, that a good seal is critical to the success of a crown or any dental restoration. The poorer the fit of the crown, the more cement will be needed; the greater the thickness of cement, the more likelihood there is of dissolution of the cement and the consequent failure of the seal. If the crown fits poorly at the margins, we will have the very undesirable situation of having a bulk of cement in this critical area. Over a period of time this cement will tend to dissolve out, leaving a leaking, unprotected margin, and making failure very likely. This is another drawback of faulty margins. Good seal can be developed by very close adaptation of the margins to the tooth, coupled with a nearly microscopic thickness of cement.

The shell crown is made by a venerable but obsolete crown-making technique that is still infrequently used by some dentists. Unlike the cast crown, which is duplicated in metal from a precise wax pattern by the lost-wax casting technique, the shell crown is swaged over a model of the tooth. Swaging is a method of forming the crown by pressing soft gold over the die. Although I have seen some good shell crowns with decent margins, the great majority had atrocious margins. The shell crown technique is difficult; it is much easier to obtain accurate results using cast crowns. Because of their poor fit, shell crowns used a large amount of cement; many of these crowns were in effect crowns of cement covered with a thin layer of soft gold. This was highly unsatisfactory from the engineering point of view; as the cement began to deteriorate, the restoration lost its support and its marginal seal. The same situation would be present in a cast crown with bad margins, though even a poorly made cast crown stands a better chance of succeeding than a shell crown with poor margins. The cast crown with poor margins will at least fit accurately against the tooth in many places and thus may provide a seal in such areas, while the shell crown with poor margins may not fit accurately anywhere. On the other hand, a well-made shell crown is vastly superior to a badly made cast crown. In this case, however, the critical difference is in workmanship, not technique. The cast crown is stronger, and the cast crown technique makes it easier to achieve good margins and close overall fit. This explains why cast crowns have been universally accepted by dentistry.

On esthetic grounds most people object to gold crowns and other metal restorations that are too conspicuous. To meet their objections, veneers, or coverings, of esthetic materials are applied to metal restorations that would be visible when the patient speaks or smiles. Veneering techniques have advanced today to a point such that the most exacting esthetic demands can be met in nearly all cases. It is important to remember, however, that the crown is *not* made of the veneering material, but of metal, usually gold, which is simply covered by the veneer. The function of the veneer is strictly esthetic; it is the metal shell which establishes the fit, the marginal adaptation, and the solid foundation of the crown.

Some of the newer veneering materials are quite strong. Dense porcelains can be baked onto high-fusing gold alloys for more esthetic results. Acrylic plastic, the most common veneering material, is being supplemented by stronger vinyl and epoxy resins with good results.

The porcelain jacket crown is an exception. Here, porcelain, ordinarily a veneering material, comprises the whole crown; there is no metal shell. Although porcelain is a fairly strong ceramic material, it is much more brittle than metal, and is susceptible to fracture. But porcelain is probably the most esthetic material that dentistry has, and it is capable of producing extremely beautiful restorations. The use of the porcelain jacket is usually restricted to the front teeth, where the need for excellent esthetics is most critical and the functional demands of heavy chewing are the least.

The preparation of a tooth for a porcelain jacket differs from the preparation for an ordinary crown in the need for a shoulder. This shoulder, which must extend completely around the tooth, is required to make room for the necessary additional bulk of material needed for strength. Impression techniques are similar to those used for metal crowns, but the manufacture of the porcelain crown is much more difficult.

Although more accurate marginal fits are possible with gold crowns than with porcelain jackets, fairly close adaptation at the margins is possible with porcelain, and a well-made jacket should not require much cement. Again, a very thin cement is most desirable. A common cause of porcelain jacket failure is seen clinically as a dark line of discoloration of the tooth at the gum line. This may indicate a poor margin and a thick mass of cement which, in time, dissolves out. Thus the seal is lost, and leakage and discoloration follow. In such cases the poor appearance of the tooth is often accentuated by a recession of the gum, possibly caused by irritation at the bad margin. Usually the only cure for such a situation is a new jacket, this time with proper margins.

Gum-line discoloration is quite common, and at times may be completely unavoidable, especially if the jacket is made when the patient is in his teens. Some recession of the gums subsequent to the teen years is quite normal. This recession may disclose a margin previously covered by the gum. At times it is possible to compensate for an expected recession by preparing the gingival margins (shoulders) fairly well under the gums. In cases where such preparation is not feasible, the margin is quite likely to be exposed after some years. A very good margin has the best chance of retaining good esthetics after gum recession, though even the best margins may not be esthetically unsatisfactory after exposure. In such cases a new jacket may be necessary.

There is no guarantee that a tooth that is crowned will be immune from further problems, though careful maintenance should minimize the risks. The care of teeth that have been restored with crowns or jackets is similar to the care necessary for any tooth. Good oral hygiene is, of course, a must; dental floss and the Water

Pik can be most helpful. Routine examinations are necessary to check on any periodontal damage or marginal decay, and continuing periodontal care is essential. In addition to the usual periodontal considerations, any gingival recession may expose the root area beyond a margin to decay. Ideally, the margin of a crown or jacket should extend just below the free margin of the gingiva so that the gum prevents the margins from collecting food debris. Recession of the gum of course exposes the margin to food debris; any subsequent slackness in matters of oral hygiene may be drastically punished by hard-to-treat decay around the margin of the crown. Such decay can make a whole new crown necessary.

American dentistry has long held the reputation of being the best in the world. Most of this reputation has been based on the beauty of our finished restorative procedures, such as crowns, jackets, and fixed bridgework. A patient fortunate enough to enjoy the benefits of such a restoration must never forget that only the most careful methods of oral hygiene will insure the longest possible service with the least trouble.

Our old friend Dr. Poorwork pops up here, since he occasionally tries his hand at "cap-work." His powerful reluctance to spend sufficient time with his patients shows up in crowns with undercut preparations, possibly with decay still present, crowns with overextended and badly adapted margins, and crowns with bulging contours and poor occlusion. A Poorwork crown can often be detected by the surrounding gums, which may be red, swollen, and oozing from the constant irritation from the badly adapted margin. Occasionally he fashions a jacket by pressing down over the tooth an acrylic shell filled with quick-setting plastic. Such a restoration is used by good dentists only as a temporary crown while the permanent jacket is being made; it cannot possibly have properly adapted margins. Yet I have seen many such jackets passed off as permanent restorations. Perhaps Dr. Poorwork should be applauded for such work, which does after all represent an improvement for him. His usual treatment for badly broken-down teeth is to extract them.

15

Root Canal

The methods of root canal treatment, or endodontia (endo = inside, dont = tooth), have come a long way since the "killing-the-nerve" treatments of old-fashioned dentistry. Today root canal procedures are so good that there is hardly ever any reason to extract a tooth because of infection or inflammation of the pulp. But despite the convincing success of carefully executed root canal procedures, most people still believe that an abscessed tooth must be extracted. This is but another of the many current erroneous notions about dentistry.

The healthy tooth has a hollow canal within the hard layers of enamel, cementum, and dentin. (For further information on the anatomy of the tooth and the function of the pulp, see the chapter On the Mouth.) This passageway consists of the root portion, or root canal, and, within the crown of the tooth, a portion

179

called the pulp chamber. The root canal and the pulp chamber of a healthy tooth are filled with a soft, highly sensitive, highly vascular, blood-filled tissue called the pulp, inaccurately known to most laymen as the "nerve." The pulp is important, as we have seen, but it can also be very troublesome.

Though it is not a nerve, the pulp is extremely painful if touched, or in response to even slight irritation. Anyone who has had a toothache can confirm that an irritated or inflamed pulp can be fantastically painful. A condition of slight irritation of the pulp is called pulpal hyperemia. Typically, hyperemic pulp is sensitive to the pressures resulting from biting and to the action of sweet or acid food juices. Hyperemia may be episodic, even coming and going, perhaps, with changes of the season. Most people can recall days when taking a cold drink, or chewing ice cream with the front teeth proved painful; on such days the teeth, or some of them, were hyperemic. On other days, when the teeth were not hyperemic, cold food or drink would not elicit a painful response. Hyperemia may be innocuous, yet it is often a stage in the development of a full-blown pulpitis, which is more than a mere irritation. As its name implies, pulpitis is an inflammation of the pulp. The pain that results from it is old-fashioned toothache, and is almost always very severe. Root canal work is always necessary in the treatment of the condition which brings on a toothache. The only alternative treatment for pulpitis is the unsatisfactory one of extracting the tooth.

Our old friend, dental decay, is the best-known cause of pulpitis. Dental caries, if untreated, relentlessly continues its course toward the pulp. The progress of decay may be fast or slow, depending on the individual and the circumstances. As the decay advances, the pulp retreats from the oncoming caries by laying down layers of secondary dentin, effectively increasing the amount of sound tooth the decay must destroy before reaching the pulp. In the end, the decay will win the race and penetrate into the pulp chamber or root canal, infecting the pulp. Like other tissue, the pulp responds to infection by becoming inflamed and by swelling. But while other tissues, such as those around a boil, have room in which to swell, the pulp, which is encased in a narrow canal surrounded by walls of hard tooth, does not. The resulting pressure builds up quickly, and soon the owner of the tooth finds himself with an excruciatingly painful toothache.

The pressure and the pain of a toothache build up until there is sufficient pressure to force the pus through the tiny hole at the apex, or very end, of the root. Depending on the type of infection, the pus that drains through the hole in the root into the soft tissues may cause generalized swelling. This leads to a dangerous condition called cellulitis which, if untreated, can have fatal consequences. The classic image of the man with the toothache—handkerchief wrapped around a swollen face—is not so funny in view of the potential outcome. Curiously, the pain of the toothache's acute phase subsides when the swelling takes place. This is because the pressure on the pulp is relieved as the pus and gases formed by the infection escape via the apical foramen (the hole in the root) into the soft tissues of the face to cause the generalized inflammation. An examination of the skulls of primitive man at the Museum of Natural History in New York shows that a number of these men suffered from massive jaw infections, which may well have caused their death. One of the larger dinosaurs shows a similar huge jaw infection.

Cellulitis can almost always be treated successfully if tackled in time. Simple surgical techniques, to establish drainage, and antibiotic therapy are used. It may seem surprising to some to learn that the offending tooth can nearly always be saved by root canal treatment.

Caries-induced pulpitis does not always lead to cellulitis; more often drainage is innocently established by way of a fistula, which is a tunnel-like opening in the tissue. The common gum boil is a stage in the development of the fistula. A fistula of this sort should be treated by cleaning up the infection in the tooth with root canal work.

Many cases of pulpitis wind up as genuine abcesses, which are areas walled-off by thickened tissue set as a body defense against the infection. Certain types of bacterial agents, such as staphylococcus, tend to produce infective lesions of the abscess type. In a pulpitis eruption of this sort, suppurative material often forces its way out of the apical foramen and localizes at the root-tip to form the abscess. In the early stages, the resulting lesion usually consists of granulation tissue, and is called a granuloma. At later stages the lesion may organize into a genuine cyst. These conditions, diagnosable by X-ray, should also be treated with root canal therapy.

The tooth usually remains very tender to the touch even after drainage has relieved the acute pain of pulpitis, and regardless of whether the result is cellulitis, a fistula, or an abscess. This tender condition is a symptom of pericementitis (per = around, cementum = root surface, itis = inflammation). Pericementitis is most often a sign of abscess or cyst formation; it can also be an indication of advanced periodontal disease.

When infected matter has not erupted through the root-end it is often extremely difficult for the dentist to tell whether a tooth with symptoms involving the pulp presents a case of pulpitis, which requires root canal work, or a case of hyperemia, which does not. X-rays may be of little help in this predicament, and various means of testing the vitality of the pulp are not always conclusive. A tooth that is *clearly* not responding to thermal or electrically induced stimuli may be considered nonvital,[1] or as having a diseased pulp, and therefore in need of root canal work, though many tests of this nature are inconclusive. An analysis of symptoms is often the best course. The accompanying table shows a differential symptomatic diagnosis of hyperemia and pulpitis. The information is elicited by testing and questioning.

Differential Symptomatic Diagnosis of Hyperemia and Pulpitis

Hyperemia	Pulpitis
1. Recurs and goes away for long periods of time.	1. Continues to develop slowly into a toothache.
2. Sensitive to cold.	2. Sensitive to hot.
3. Relieved by warmth.	3. Relieved by cold.
4. No pain on tapping the tooth (no pericementitis).	4. Pain on tapping (pericementitis).
5. No aching independent of stimuli.	5. Independent aching, particularly at night or while lying down.
6. No stinging pain with chewing.	6. Pain with chewing.

---

[1] Nonvital does not mean dead. The pulp of a nonvital tooth that has not been treated has lost its vitality; the *nonvital pulp* of such a tooth must be removed with root canal treatment. But a nonvital tooth is *itself* anything but a dead tooth. Properly treated with root canal therapy, the nonvital tooth probably has as good a chance of remaining in good health as a vital tooth, which has a healthy, functioning pulp. A tooth that has been treated endodontically is nonvital, but it is not dead.

These are only characteristic pain patterns, and of course are subject to many variations. For example, a hyperemic tooth may produce a severe throbbing ache after exposure to cold, while ordinarily a throbbing ache would tend to indicate pulpitis. Once a careful diagnosis of pulpitis is established, treatment should be instituted at once.

There are other causes of pulpitis besides caries. Any severe trauma can cause irreversible damage to the pulp and start it on its way to a pulpitis. This path may include a stage of hyperemia lasting even for many years before pulpitis finally develops; when it comes it may be so remote in time from the original injury that the cause has been forgotten. Overheating, a physical blow, trauma caused by extensive use of a dental drill, unsuccessful partial endodontic procedures, such as pulp-capping or pulpotomy, or even deep decay apparently successfully treated, can all traumatize the pulp so severely that years later a pulpitis will develop.

Severe periodontal disease can also lead to an infected pulp. When bone has been lost to the level of the apex of one of the roots of a multirooted tooth, periodontal infection may enter the tooth through the apical foramen and attack the pulp from this "backwards" direction. Cases of this sort are difficult to treat; though success is usually achieved by a combination of endodontic and periodontal procedures, failure is not uncommon.

Root canal treatment most often is treatment of the disease inside the individual tooth. This involves cleaning out the root canal, establishing drainage of infection through the root canal, widening the canal to prepare for a filling, establishing control of infection and absolute sterility of the canal, and finally filling and sealing the canal with a sterile, tight filling. The idea is to clear up the infection and then to replace the removed pulp with a tightly sealed filling so that the infection will not recur.

In endodontia as in most areas of dentistry there is general agreement on aims, but not on methods. Here is a brief outline of a commonly accepted root canal technique:

1. A hole is drilled in the tooth to obtain access to the root canal. Pus may pour from a freshly tapped root canal, and a patient in great pain often experiences dramatic relief as the drainage reduces the pressure inside the tooth.
2. The canal is now penetrated with small, needle-shaped files and other instruments, and the pulp is utterly removed. Often there is little left of the pulp but a strand of shriveled tissue, or a glob of putrescent matter. All material must ultimately be removed from the canal. The canal is widened by filing with successively larger files. Before this widening is accomplished, the exact length of the canal must be ascertained by taking an X-ray with a file in place, and rechecking the measurement until it is exact. During the widening process, the canal is flushed and cleaned by irrigating with water and chemical agents; double-strength chlorinated soda is a popular and effective agent for this. When the canal is sufficiently widened, it is flushed again and dried. Needle-like absorbent paper points are placed within the canal to blot it dry. A dressing can now be placed within the canal by moistening a paper point with a strong sterilizing agent and leaving the medicated point within the canal for a few days. The idea is to establish drainage of any periapical (around-the-root-tip) infection through the apical foramen, and thence through

the root canal, and at the same time to combat the infection with chemical agents. To allow for easier drainage, the canal is often left open at this stage. At a subsequent visit the canal is again flushed, dried, and remedicated, and then it is sealed tightly by plugging the access hole in the tooth.

3. These procedures of flushing, drying, medicating, and sealing are repeated at subsequent visits until the dentist is satisfied that the canal is clean and sterile. Many dentists use bacteriological cultures to verify sterility. The root canal is now filled and sealed. Gutta percha is considered by many to be the best material for the root canal filling. It is a tacky, inert substance which, when sealed with chloropercha, itself a mixture of gutta percha and chloroform, and tightly packed, provides an excellent seal. Gutta percha can also be used with many other sealing agents. In thin, tortuous canals in which gutta percha cannot easily be handled, silver points, with sealers, are used as the root canal filling. When the root canal has been filled and sealed, the tooth is ready for a functional restoration — a filling, crown, or whatever.

For a variety of reasons, endodontic work is sometimes done on vital teeth that show no signs of puplitis. If a necessary restorative procedure requires cutting a tooth down to the pulp, root canal work is usually done. Sometimes the root canal of a vital tooth is needed as anchorage for a restoration; perhaps removal of deep decay involves the pulp and the dentist feels that immediate root canal will fare better than pulp-capping or pulpotomy (see below).

Root canal work is done on vital teeth for all these

reasons, and for others. There is no concern with infection in the case of a vital tooth, so many dentists complete the entire root canal procedure on such teeth in one visit.

The treatment and filling of root canals are not the only methods of endodontic treatment. There are minor endodontic procedures which are easier and less costly than root canal, but which can be successfully employed only on selected vital teeth. But nonvital teeth in adults *always* require root canal work.

Pulp-capping is the most popular of these minor endodontic procedures. It occasionally happens, after a tooth is completely cleaned of caries, that the dentist sees a pulpal exposure, or unintentional opening into the pulp chamber, where the pulp is visible. If the exposure is clean, pulp-capping can be tried. The tooth is isolated from saliva by a rubber-dam or cotton-roll technique, and it is cleaned, most often with hydrogen peroxide. The exposure is dried and covered with a preparation containing calcium hydroxide. The tooth is then treated with sedative materials and filled. Treatment may extend to more than one visit. The key to the treatment is the action of the calcium hydroxide, a caustic substance which, over a period of time, often stimulates the pulp to form secondary dentin and thus bridge the exposure.

If the pulp in the pulp chamber, when it is exposed to view, is seen not to be clean, but it is likely that the root canal is not yet involved, then a pulpotomy, or partial removal of the pulp, can be tried. It is my experience that both pulp-capping and pulpotomy, when carefully done, will deliver excellent results. In pulpotomy, the pulp in the pulp chamber is removed with a bur or other instrument, the opening is flooded with peroxide until the bleeding is brought under control, the calcium hydroxide preparation is used, and the procedure is continued as in pulp-capping. If either pulp-capping or pulpotomy fail, then root canal therapy still can be done. All in all, the high degree of success with the various methods of endodontia are largely responsible for the modern dentist's claim that extractions are almost never necessary.

In certain extreme cases, where a root-end infection persists despite treatment, an apicoectomy can be tried (apico = apex, ectomy = cut out). An apicoectomy is a surgical removal of the apex of the root with the surrounding persistent infection, whether an abcess, granuloma, or cyst. The gum is incised at the level of the root-tip, the thin outer bone layer is removed, exposing the apex of the root, the surrounding tissue is cleaned of infection with surgical curettes, a few millimeters of the root-tip are cut off, the apex is sealed, often with silver amalgam, and the area is sutured. Usually the root canal filling is made at the same time. This procedure, less complicated than it sounds, has succeeded when all else has failed.

In common with all other forms of dentistry, endodontic work can be done poorly, carelessly, and hastily. Many people believe that an endodontically treated tooth will turn black. While this often happens to badly treated teeth, it is the experience of good dentists that teeth do not turn black following careful endodontic treatment. Teeth will discolor following root canal treatment when diseased pulp is not thoroughly cleaned out, when the root canal is not sterilized, when decay remains in the crown of the tooth; in short, when a hasty, sloppy job is done. Dr. Poorwork, when he bothers to do root canal work at all, has his own methods, which are predicated on the amount of time he is willing to spend, that is to say, very little. Often the infected tooth is opened and the pulp chemically devitalized. This relieves the pain, but often does little to control the infection, with the result that the tooth is lost. Dr. Poorwork often follows up his chemical treatment with a half-hearted root canal filling that does not extend to the proper length. For years such treatment was known to laymen as "killing the nerve," and that's about the size of it. Still, such perfunctory treatment sometimes meets with some success when nature does most of the healing work. Even so, teeth so treated are likely to discolor, and may at last have to be extracted.

16

Oral Surgery

The letters "D.D.S." after a dentist's name stand for "doctor of dental surgery." All dentists are surgeons, and all dental procedures are surgical procedures in that they involve the manipulation and instrumentation of tissue. Nevertheless, "oral surgery" has come to mean surgical procedures other than those which serve to treat and restore lesions of the teeth. As a rule, oral surgery is surgery involving bone and gums as well as teeth. Although all dentists have had training in such surgery, there are many oral surgical procedures which call for more specialized facilities than those of the typical dental office. Many oral surgical procedures, furthermore, are beyond the range of experience of most general practitioners. It is for these reasons that the specialty of oral surgery has developed.

Exodontia (from the Greek exo = out, dont = tooth) is that branch of dentistry that deals with the

190

extraction of teeth, and it is the extraction of teeth which comprises the great bulk of the work of oral surgeons, who are also called exodontists. All dentists are trained to do the simpler surgical procedures, which include the great majority of tooth extractions, but many dentists refer patients needing an extraction to an exodontist. Usually this is because the dentist prefers to avoid the bother and possible complications of extractions, and because he knows that the exodontist is better equipped and better trained to perform such work. It is uncommon that the patients of a good dentist require extractions anyway, and he may not want to equip his office for procedures that are relatively rare in his practice.

Although extractions make up most of the volume of practice of an oral surgeon, most of his special training and study has dealt with operations much less frequently called for, and which the average general practitioner will not tackle. Among these are operations for impacted teeth; the reduction of jaw fractures; sinus operations; the removal of tumors of the mouth, head, and neck; and the removal of retained broken-root tips, salivary-gland stones, and bone irregularities.

Of all the oral-surgery procedures, the extraction of teeth is the one with which the layman is the most familiar. An extraction is ordinarily a relatively simple affair, particularly by comparison with the work required to restore a tooth. The typical extraction, including anesthesia and assuming careful, cautious instrumentation, may take five or ten minutes at most, and is without incident. Excluding the waiting period required for the anesthesia to take effect, the average time required to pull a typical tooth is perhaps one minute. It is a quick and easy job, which hardly taxes the skill or stamina of an experienced practitioner.

But things can and occasionally do go wrong, and here is where the oral surgeon should be summoned.

During the course of an extraction a root or tip of a root may break off and remain in the jaw. The dentist should check the extracted tooth for signs of a broken root tip. If a root or tip has broken, it must not be left in the jaw, where it would be a potential source of infection or cyst formation. If the dentist is unable to remove the tip, he should explain the situation, which is certainly not uncommon, and at once refer the case to an oral surgeon. Leaving the root in, in the hope that nothing will come of it, is extremely bad practice. But some dentists are reluctant to refer a case involving a retained root tip to a specialist, because they fear the patient may think them incompetent. One of the reasons for taking complete X-rays of toothless patients before making full dentures is to discover retained root tips. It is often desirable to remove these before making the dentures. In some cases, depending upon the circumstances, it may be preferable to leave a deeply imbedded root tip alone if it is not infected or a source of pathology.

A root tip broken off during extraction is likely to be sterile, and it is therefore less likely to give trouble than the remaining tip of a tooth that has rotted away. Some tips are retained not as a result of improper or incomplete surgery, but are simply all that is left of a rotted tooth. Sometimes the gums will even grown over such a root tip. Because of the decayed material around the lesion, a root tip of this sort is never sterile, and, if not already a source of infection, is very likely to cause trouble in the future. In these cases it is nearly always desirable to remove the root tip.

Removal of an impacted tooth is a job which few general practitioners are willing to tackle, and which most often is referred to the oral surgeon. An impacted tooth is one which is "stuck"; it has somehow been blocked as it attempted to erupt. One common cause of impactions is the premature removal of baby teeth, resulting in a shifting of position of one or two of the remaining teeth into the area in which the permanent tooth should erupt. As the permanent tooth tries to move into position, it is blocked by the adjacent teeth, which have moved too close together. (See chapter on The Care of Children's Teeth.) Such an impacted tooth is usually a problem for the orthodontist, who tries to move the adjacent teeth apart, thereby allowing enough room for the impacted tooth to move into position. Occasionally the oral surgeon is asked to help, sometimes by removing bone which has formed and thickened around the impacted tooth and further blocks its eruption. In cases that cannot be remedied orthodontically, the oral surgeon is asked to remove the impacted tooth.

The most common teeth to become impacted are the third molars, or wisdom teeth. The wisdom tooth, like the appendix, is a vestigial organ. Man today has smaller jaws, but as many teeth as his antecedents. The result is that, for most people, there is not enough room in the mouth for the wisdom teeth; they have no function but to give trouble, and there are many cases of people who do not grow wisdom teeth. Occasionally dentists see a person with a fourth molar, or second wisdom tooth. This does not mean that such a person is a throwback to the apes any more than an individual who never had wisdom teeth can be accounted an evolutionary advance. The phenomenon simply demonstrates that the wisdom teeth, being vestigial, are subject to variations in number. Variations in size and shape are also common; many people have irregularly shaped wisdom teeth, especially uppers, with tiny roots.

The wisdom teeth usually begin to appear between the ages of fifteen and twenty-five. If the jaws are not large enough for them to fit neatly into the dental arch, the teeth will not erupt normally and will become impacted.

Jawbone irregularities sometimes lessen the chances of making comfortable, functional dentures. Alveolectomy is the name given to a popular operation in which the edges of the jawbone, or alveolar bone, are trimmed to give a better seat for the dentures. Some patients have a torus, which is a healthy if somewhat uncommon lump of bone, harmless in itself, that greatly complicates the making of dentures. It may therefore have to be removed before dentures are constructed. Occasionally people whose bony structure is too thin and meagre to give decent support to a denture can be helped surgically. One treatment being tried with some success is a lengthening of the effective surface of the bony ridge by surgically deepening the fold of the lip in the direction of the angle of the jaw.

Although the oral surgeon is a true specialist who has had years of additional training, he may find himself in the paradoxical position of being a specialist acting as a technician, having his diagnoses performed for him by a referring dentist or, often, even by the patient. Frequently the oral surgeon receives a patient from a referring dentist, with instructions to extract a certain tooth or teeth. Naturally, the surgeon performs the requested procedure. Nor is it uncommon for a patient who has not been referred to point to a tooth and say to the oral surgeon, "This one hurts," in the expectation that it will be extracted. At this, most oral surgeons shrug their shoulders and extract the tooth. In doing so, in effect, they act like mechanics or technicians, rather than as doctors. They do not use their knowledge to establish a diagnosis and proper course of treatment, but merely follow someone else's prescription.

Most teeth that are extracted could have been saved by modern dental treatment. Of course the oral surgeon knows this as well as any dentist does, and here we discover an interesting ethical question. When a patient with a toothache comes in for an extraction will the oral surgeon try to talk him out of having the tooth pulled? Will the oral surgeon take the time to establish a proper diagnosis and then explain that the tooth can be saved, for example with root canal work, followed by a major restoration, none of which work he performs himself? Or will he shrug his shoulders, extract the tooth, and collect the fee? The profession of oral surgery is beset by the paradox that a man who is highly trained and skilled should spend most of his time doing extractions, which are relatively menial work, which he rarely prescribes himself, and which, in most cases, should not even be performed, being in fact the least preferred treatment for the patient. Curiously, most surgeons have come to terms with this problem without disturbing their philosophic equilibrium.

17

Orthodontia

As the general level of prosperity has risen over the past several years an increasing number of parents have decided that they want their children to enjoy the advantages of "straight teeth, a nice smile, and a good bite." The result has been a skyrocketing increase in the popularity of orthodontic treatment, which is an attempt to correct or stabilize the position of the teeth, usually through the use of adjustable braces. Most of the patients are children, but the treatment of adults is occasionally feasible. Although some general practitioners do orthodontic work, the great bulk of it is done by specialists who limit their practices to orthodontia. It is a lucrative field.

Orthodontia is one of the most controversy-ridden of dental disciplines. Cases for which one school of orthodontists prescribes a certain type of treatment are analyzed and treated in an entirely different fashion by another school. Treatment that is accepted as standard practice by one group is condemned by another. There are no convincing statistics to demonstrate the superiority of one method over another, and there may never be, because it is so hard to isolate and evaluate all the variables. It is in such a theoretical climate that orthodontia is practiced, and there is no hope of resolving the controversies soon. Thus the practice of orthodontia is today more of an art than a science.

How many children need orthodontic work? Cynics have said that the orthodontic need of a child is in direct proportion to his parents' ability to pay. It is true that almost everyone has something less than a perfect bite, but it does not follow that most people need orthodontic treatment. A slight imperfection in the alignment of the front teeth is in itself insufficient reason for orthodontic treatment. Many parents, terrified that they may not be doing everything they should for their child, actually do him a disservice when they arrange for unnecessary orthodontic work, and many orthodontists are too willing to accept patients who do not need their attention. The criteria for a normal bite include both esthetic and functional considerations. If the appearance is not adversely affected, and the bite is comfortable, and chewing is efficient, and there are no stresses on the teeth that might result in periodontal damage, then there is no need for orthodontic therapy. But there are Poorworks in orthodontia, too, and there is always a chance that one of them may recommend treatment when none is needed. The best guide to the integrity of the orthodontist is the patient's conscientious dentist, who is in a position to evaluate the specialist's way of working.

In the typical child, the development of the dentition

follows certain normal patterns that eventually lead to a normal adult dentition with a normal occlusion. The normal dentition is any dentition that is within acceptable limits of function and appearance. As the teeth erupt and take their place in the developing dental arch, the growth and development of the jawbone keep pace with and are profoundly affected by the eruption and positioning of the teeth. (The chapter on The Care of Children's Teeth contains more detail on this process.) If for any reason some teeth are prevented from taking their correct positions in the arch, the whole developmental mechanism of the jaws can be upset, often with unpleasant results for the formation of the face and profile. Preventive and corrective orthodontic work, by effecting better positioning of the teeth, often improves the development of the jaw and thus leads to greatly improved appearance.

In many cases the results of orthodontic treatment are dramatic. A child whose facial appearance is marred by a faulty dentition may show an astounding improvement in appearance as relatively simple orthodontic treatment progresses. Dramatic changes in profile and facial form often accompany the realignment of the teeth. Favorable results of this sort have the most positive effect on the child's developing personality; it is no exaggeration to say that effective orthodontic therapy can profoundly affect the whole subsequent life experience. Perhaps it is the realization of this fact which makes people willing to pay the high fees of the orthodontist.

That this repositioning of the teeth can be effected at all depends on the unique properties of the alveolar bone of the jaws. The alveolar bone is that part of the jawbone which directly surrounds the roots of the teeth. Pressure in certain directions, applied through the teeth to the alveolar bone, results in a resorption of the bone, an actual dissolution; the bone elements are decalcified and carried off by the bloodstream. Yet force applied to the alveolar bone in *other* directions can serve to strengthen it. These properties of alveolar bone can cause problems in adult life; resorption of the bone as a result of certain pressures, including those of malocclusion, leads to periodontal disease. Often an important part of periodontal treatment is a reshaping of the teeth to eliminate destructive pressures on the bone. But careful exploitation of the special responses of alveolar bone enables the orthodontist to relocate the teeth of children. By the use of braces, the orthodontist creates a *controlled* pressure that causes a *controlled* resorption of the alveolar bone. As the bone is resorbed in response to the pressures from the appliances, the tooth, guided by the appliance, moves into the space created by the resorption. If the patient is young, and assuming the forces have not been excessive, then new alveolar bone grows in behind the tooth, to fill the space that has been vacated. This explains how the orthodontist can seem to move a tooth bodily through a block of solid bone.

The genuine need for orthodontic treatment is widespread, and the causes of this need are many. One of the commonest causes of an occlusal defect requiring orthodontic correction is the premature loss of baby teeth. (See chapter on The Care of Children's Teeth.) Certain habits of childhood sometimes cause malocclusions that call for orthodontic treatment. Thumb-sucking may leave a child with a classical pattern of anterior arch deformation; this condition generally corrects itself when the habit is broken, provided it is broken early enough. Pencil-chewing, teddy-bear chewing, and so on, and certain habitual movements of cheek, lip, and tongue are capable of producing the sort of persistent pressures on the teeth that may cause them to shift. This is not to suggest that all such habits are necessarily harmful to the dentition; in fact, great numbers of children go through a stage of thumb-sucking, and so on, without any harm being done to the teeth. Still, the potential for damage is there, and sometimes it is realized.

There are many approaches to breaking these habits. Sometimes applied child psychology is used to discourage them; sometimes appliances are constructed to block the physical movements associated with the habits; sometimes vile-tasting chemicals are placed on the finger that is sucked. The best approach is to consider the exact habits, personality, and needs of the individual child before taking steps to break or divert the habit. Some authorities have suggested that pacifiers may lead to trouble with the dentition, but it is my feeling that these devices can be used as long as there is no definite evidence of a developing malocclusion. If such evidence is present, it's time to see the dentist.

A program for prevention of malocclusion in a child calls for good care of the primary teeth, so that none are lost ahead of time, and the discovery, analysis, and correction of harmful habits. If a baby tooth is lost prematurely, it is usually good practice to employ a space-maintainer. This appliance maintains the space vacated by the lost tooth and thus keeps the other teeth in their proper places until the permanent tooth is ready to erupt. Destructive habits may be harder to handle. But malocclusion cannot necessarily be prevented by even the most enlightened actions of parent and dentist. Whenever malocclusion arises, whether through neglect or despite the best preventive measures, orthodontic treatment may be advisable.

In such cases the first step is to discuss things with

the family dentist, who may find that there is really no problem after all. The new front teeth rarely come in straight, and I have had to reassure many a panicky parent that they would straighten themselves out as the jaw develops. When the family dentist does spot a potential malocclusion he will be the best one to judge whether a consultation with an orthodontist is in order. If treatment is recommended, and the parent is concerned about fees, frank discussions with the orthodontist and the family dentist may help the parent decide whether the benefits will be worth their cost.

The controversies between orthodontists never seem to let up. In recent years the use of the extra-oral headcap appliance has again become popular with many practitioners, though the same device is still condemned by other orthodontists who believe it may cause skull deformities, among other things. Some orthodontists believe that certain malocclusions are best treated by extracting certain teeth, while others violently condemn all extraction techniques. One school of orthodontists uses appliances which expand the dental arches to make room for badly positioned teeth; other orthodontists claim that most expansion cases tend to relapse. And so the arguments rage. Since I lack the qualifications of an orthodontist, I will refrain from adding my own voice to the general clamor. Suffice it to say here that most orthodontic treatment is relatively successful, since most experienced orthodontists are sufficiently flexible to select, in each instance, a course of treatment suited to the particular demands of the case.

There are possible drawbacks to orthodontia, and a parent contemplating treatment for his child ought to be aware of them. First of all, there is no assurance that the treatment will be successful. Even apparently successful treatment sometimes relapses in a few years to the old malocclusion. To head off a relapse, a minority of patients have to wear a retainer appliance at night. Sometimes orthodontic treatment damages the teeth and alveolar bone. Teeth that are moved too quickly, with too much force, may be weakened by having part of their roots resorbed; occasionally such teeth become devitalized. Sometimes orthodontic treatment brings little improvement. With the occlusion still not functionally efficient, the patient is then a candidate for later periodontal difficulties, just as he was beforehand. But all in all, the potential benefits of needed orthodontic treatment far outweigh the possible drawbacks.

The careful orthodontist keeps in mind a number of precautions that he will wish to take during the course of treatment. Bands made around the teeth for the support and anchorage of braces should be made to fit snugly, and they should be carefully cemented, to prevent decay under the bands. But even a well-made appliance is an efficient food collector, and unless it is kept clean it may become an indirect cause of decay. The patient should therefore be given full instructions on keeping his appliances clean. At intervals in treatment the orthodontist may remove all appliances in order to permit the family dentist to check for decay. Intelligent cooperation between parent, specialist, and dentist provides the best chance to realize the full potential benefits of orthodontic treatment.

There are not nearly enough orthodontists to meet the need for treatment. In the future we may see the expanded use of trained orthodontic technicians who, though not dentists, would be qualified to perform certain orthodontic procedures: taking impressions, making bands, cementing and adjusting bands, repairs, laboratory procedures, and simple adjustments of appliances. Freed of this technical work, the orthodontist could concentrate on the planning, design, diagnosis, and supervision of cases; thus he could handle a great many more cases. Such expansion of the effective orthodontic manpower might also help bring fees down to more reasonable levels.

18

Cosmetic Dentistry

Throughout history, man's vanity has led him to make sacrifices for the sake of his appearance without regard to the consequences for his health. Though modern dentistry should not lend its name or services to such folly, there is, at least in the public's eye, such a thing as "cosmetic dentistry." This concept is encouraged by some dentists who, mindful of the money to be made by an appeal to human vanity, may actually like to think of themselves as cosmeticians. Yet cosmetic dentistry is not a legitimate branch of dental practice, and it is unfortunate that there should even be such a term. The dentist is properly a healer, not a beautician.

The public has some curious notions on the subject of dental cosmetics. It is generally believed that a beautiful smile can be obtained by "capping" the teeth, and many people have been dissuaded from having their teeth capped for this purpose only by the high cost involved. Many believe that the first thing a would-be starlet must do is have her teeth capped, and that every resident of Hollywood sports plastic teeth. Some think that capping the teeth will protect them from future trouble, and many believe that there are dentists who "specialize" in cosmetic dentistry. Perhaps these people believe it is beyond the capability of the regular dentist to do a good-looking, cosmetic job, and that somehow the secret of attractive dentistry reposes with some so-called cosmetic dentists, whoever they may be.

These curiously popular ideas are nonsense. The truth is that this type of work is not to be taken lightly, that it represents major expenditures of time and money, and, most important, that it constitutes *major* dental surgery. It often involves the removal of a large bulk of tooth tissue from a great many teeth. Consequently it is work that should be prescribed and undertaken only for grave and sufficient reasons. A somewhat crooked tooth is not reason enough.

What may be involved in a so-called cosmetic dental restoration? Of course, all dental restorations are cosmetic in the sense that the dentist considers the factor of appearance before planning the restoration. Anterior, or front-of-the-mouth, fillings provide a case in point. Although metal fillings are stronger, more esthetic plastic or silicate materials are used for up-front fillings. Moreover, an anterior filling is usually prepared from the back side of the tooth, so that the filling material, esthetic though it might be, will still show as little as possible. But even a mouth full of conventional dental restorations, such as fillings, inlays, and crowns, will give quite a pleasing appearance for any ordinary social need; it is rare that a mouth is subjected to intense, close-up scrutiny by anybody other than a dentist.

A restoration that is done primarily for esthetic

purposes is one that might be called a cosmetic restoration. Such a restoration might involve porcelain jackets or full crowns on the six upper anterior teeth, or on both the upper and lower front teeth, or perhaps on all the front teeth and the first or the first two premolar teeth, or, in extreme cases, on every tooth in the mouth. Certainly it would be the height of extravagant vanity to have all the teeth done for cosmetic reasons alone. In the chapters on Bridgework and Crowns and Jackets I have detailed the procedures necessary to make such restorations. Those who read these passages should be impressed with the vast amount of work necessary in the preparation of such restorations, and they should be particularly impressed with the heavy bulk of tooth structure that must be cut down for crown and jacket preparations. The large amount of tooth tissue that is cut away is irreplaceable, and a crown is therefore a drastic dental measure.

The primary purpose of a crown is to restore a badly broken-down and decayed tooth that could not be satisfactorily restored with a conventional filling. Another legitimate function of a crown is to serve as a bridge abutment, or as a connection for a splint. But crowns *can* fail; dentists see many that did not succeed. Perhaps most crowns that fail do so because they were poorly done; bad margins, poor contour, incorrect occlusion are common causes of crown failure. But even a perfect crown can fail. Gingival recession can make the crowned tooth susceptible to caries. Poor oral hygiene may cause a good crown to fail under circumstances in which the intact natural tooth would not be adversely affected.

All in all, a good crown is more susceptible to failure than is an intact natural tooth, and a poor crown infinitely more so. If a filling fails, the tooth can often be salvaged with a crown. If a crown fails, another crown or perhaps a post-crown may save the tooth, though some crown failures are irreparable. A decayed tooth can be filled, and then filled again if it decays on a different surface. If the decay recurs persistently, a crown can always be made *as the method of last resort.* But when an otherwise sound tooth has already had a great bulk of material ground from it to prepare it for a merely esthetic crown, we are starting with the last resort. I have seen many of these large cosmetic restorations crumbling in the mouth after a number of years. They had to be completely redone, and occasionally teeth were lost. There is no doubt that intact natural teeth hold up much better than even the best cosmetic crown or jacket restoration, and there is no question that anything less than the best in crown or jacket work significantly multiplies the chances of failure. Anyone contemplating a major dental restoration for strictly cosmetic purposes should think twice about all these considerations.

The removal of bulk tooth structure incident to crown preparation is a definite drawback of the crown as a dental restoration. This disadvantage is very small when the tooth is already badly broken down and decayed, since it has already lost much of its substance to decay. When the tooth in question is going to be used as an abutment for a bridge or splint, then the advantages of making the crown greatly outweigh the disadvantages. But when a tooth is to be cut down for a crown whose only purpose is to correct a minor defect in appearance, then the slight advantage of making such a crown must be carefully weighed against the negative effect of cutting down an intact tooth. One does not chop off a freckled arm to replace it with a non-freckled false limb, nor does one peel off the skin of a nicotine-stained finger and wear flesh-colored gloves forever afterwards. Short-range considerations of appearance should not take precedence over long-range considerations of health and, incidentally, appearance.

A newly made cosmetic job may be an immediate esthetic improvement over the patient's natural teeth, but in ten years, if the restoration breaks down or the gums recede, exposing margins and cement lines which are discoloring, the patient may well wish he had his old natural dentition back.

There may be exceptional situations which cry for a cosmetic approach. Once in a long while one sees a mouth of intact, functional, natural teeth that are so poorly positioned and discolored as to be unsightly; in such cases a strictly cosmetic restoration would be justified. But the great majority of cases of unsightly anterior teeth are caused by plain old dental decay. In many of these cases the teeth have been filled and refilled with larger and progressively larger anterior fillings, usually silicate cement fillings, which tend to "wash out," and do not have the longevity of other types of filling materials. If these fillings have not been carefully done, and particularly if any decay has been left under the restoration, the margins may seriously discolor, and the edges of the fillings may look bluish-black through a translucent surface. Such an ugly result is quite common for the patients of Dr. Poorwork. But even the most carefully done anterior fillings may in time tend to wash out and discolor at the edges; a poor job will discolor much faster and more seriously. A front tooth looking like this is *not* a healthy tooth, and it usually retains little of its original crown tissue. As in the case of any such badly broken down tooth, the restoration of choice is a crown or jacket.

If the patient's front teeth are all so involved, as is often the case, then a series of jackets is the logical prescription. This also holds true, of course, for badly decayed front teeth that have never been filled. A series of anterior jackets made for a patient with front teeth disfigured by decay or old fillings can produce a very beautiful result, but I would not call such a case a cosmetic restoration, because the restoration was required for functional reasons, and not just for appearance. That the work looks beautiful is no reason to call the case cosmetic, nor should it be any reason for surprise. All dental work done by capable dentists should be esthetic in appearance. The difference is that even as good dentistry strives to maintain or improve the appearance, it places its primary emphasis on function. What has come to be called cosmetic dentistry, however, considers appearance first, often at the expense of function and long-range health and appearance.

A curious mystique has evolved concerning rehabilitation dentistry. One hears talk of enormous fees and "saved" mouths, and phrases like "capping service." One hears stories of elegant, elusive dentists in gold-plated offices with futuristic machinery and of a corps of beautiful and superhumanly efficient nurses. One gets the impression that the patient is fed mouth-first into a massive computerized dental machine, out of which he will inevitably emerge with a glowingly healthy mouth and a Cary Grant profile. One even hears tales of dentists who guarantee their work forever as the logical culmination of all these supermodern happenings.

There is no doubt that an attractive, well-run office with an efficient staff contributes to the patient's sense of well-being and confidence, but he must remember that he is not being fed into a machine, and that ultimately a living dentist, and no one else, is going to deal with him. In the end, all that will matter will be the work performed and the time spent by this dentist; nothing else will count. I understand that some dentists

actually do give so-called guarantees, but the idea of
a guarantee on a health service, which must be of uncertain outcome, is absurd; it is almost as if a surgeon
guaranteed the outcome of an operation. If it failed,
would the patient press his claim from the grave? And
how might the surgeon make good on his guarantee?
If a "guaranteed mouth reconstruction" were to fail,
as many do, how should the patient seek restitution?

Ethical considerations in dentistry and medicine are
sometimes complex, and cosmetic dentistry is quite
interesting in its ethical aspects. Suppose a young girl
is convinced that she would be made more attractive
and popular by a cosmetic restoration a la Hollywood,
while the dentist knows that her teeth give her a fine,
healthy, attractive appearance despite one or two teeth
being a wee bit out of line. Suppose a matron, worried
about her advancing years and proliferating wrinkles,
fixes upon the appearance of her healthy teeth and,
imagining that they are getting darker, asks the dentist
to make them white again with "caps." Suppose a man,
hit by life's frustrations and desiring a change, asks
the dentist to accommodate him with a "new smile."
Suppose any number of cases in which, for reasons of
emotion or vanity, a patient requests a merely cosmetic
job that the dentist knows to be functionally unnecessary, if not actually unsound. Just what are the dentist's ethical responsibilities?

I strongly believe that a patient should be made
aware of all the drawbacks and possible pitfalls before
any cosmetic restoration is planned. If the dentist
decides that the restoration is ill-advised or unnecessary from the functional point of view, he must tell the
patient just what he thinks. If he does not—if the patient is not made thoroughly aware of every possibility
and consideration—then the dentist has not done his
duty. I believe, furthermore, that the dentist who even
slightly encourages the patient to go ahead with an

unsound cosmetic restoration is guilty of flagrantly unethical behavior.

I have heard many dentists rationalize cosmetic dentistry that they have done at the patient's request. It has been said that one must do what the patient wants, lest the patient be antagonized and simply has the work done by another dentist. I have heard it said that it might be emotionally damaging to a patient to be told the truth, which is that the expectations of a sufficiently dramatic change in appearance and personality could not be realized by the cosmetic restoration. I have been told that such a restoration can constitute valuable psychological therapy for an anxious patient, whose hopes of a new life and new appearance should be carefully nurtured. I even remember, with a shudder, a dentist saying to me, "If the patient wants this, why shouldn't I make it? We are not God!"

I would be more moved by such pious declamations if I were not aware of the money involved. Perhaps it is not right to play God, especially when it will mean losing a high fee. Suppose a young girl comes for treatment, and the dentist, upon examination, discovers that she can be treated satisfactorily and very esthetically with a few carefully made anterior fillings, at a cost of under fifty dollars. But the girl thinks there is something wrong with her appearance and that a capping job is necessary. The dentist knows that his fee for the cosmetic restoration will be perhaps twenty times the fee for the superior treatment. He also knows that her mother wears expensive furs. Might this be a factor in his diagnosis and prescription? Will the dentist's desire to earn more money encourage him to give the girl a major restoration, which will weaken the teeth, and that may look terrible ten years hence, rather than the simpler and very superior treatment that would probably look much better than the costly job in years to come?

PART 4

ARTIFICIAL TEETH

False teeth have a history going back to ancient times. Artificial teeth roughly fashioned of wood have been found in Egyptian tombs, and one royal mummy has been reported whose mouth contained a full denture, with a base, or plate, of wood, and metal buttons for teeth. An Etruscan tomb dating back to 500 B.C. contained a bridge of ox teeth held together by gold rings. In the literature of the Romans there are many mentions of various types of false-tooth appliances, while the Talmud mentions false teeth in women, but never in men. It seems likely that, in ancient times, the chief motive for wearing what must have been ill-fitting and uncomfortable appliances was mainly esthetic. Did the typical craftsman who made these false teeth promise his customers, or patients, that his product would give their mouths sex appeal?

The branch of modern dentistry that deals with false

teeth is known as prosthetics. (Broadly speaking, however, prosthetics is the art of replacing *any* missing part of the body with an artificial structure.) To many laymen, and, alas, many dentists, prosthetics is the most important part of dentistry. This emphasis reflects an unhealthy attitude; the stress should always be on preventive and restorative work which, when properly executed, would limit prosthetics to accident cases. But it is obvious that anything so nearly ideal is far in the future. We will continue to need prosthetics for the millions as long as dentistry continues to fail in its first mission, which is to save teeth rather than to replace them.

A prosthesis, or denture, may replace one of any number of teeth. Partial dentures, to replace only some of the teeth, may be removable or fixed, or they may even contain a combination of removable and fixed elements. Full dentures are always removable.

Some people have the notion that it is the dental technician who "makes" the teeth or the restoration. This is not true. It is the dentist who makes the restoration. The dentist diagnoses, plans, designs, checks at various stages, fits, and adjusts the restoration. The technician, working in the dental laboratory, assists the dentist by performing certain of the technical procedures, tasks which are done according to the specific directions of the dentist and which the dentist has no time to do himself.

19

The Removable
Partial Denture

The commonest of all tooth replacements is the removable partial prosthesis (or bridge, or denture), most often called simply the "partial." When some teeth are present and some missing, the partial may be used to replace the missing teeth. When all the teeth are gone, the full denture must be used.

The partial is enormously popular. Indeed, it is too popular, since it is used in so many cases where a fixed bridge would serve better. Often, the key factors that cause a partial to be selected over fixed bridgework are the greater difficulty and much higher cost involved in the construction of the fixed bridge. Then, too, there are many instances in which it is not possible to make a fixed bridge; in such cases a partial is the only solution. But where an option does exist, the fixed bridge is nearly always theoretically better than the removable partial. And yet the partial that is properly prepared and constructed can be an excellent restoration.

The common word *bridge,* as used in dentistry, means just that. A space or gap in the dental arch, caused by the extraction of one or more teeth, is bridged by the appliance. The bridge goes from one tooth, over the gap, to another tooth, just as the George Washington Bridge goes from New York to New Jersey. The teeth at each end of the span that are used for support of the bridge are the abutment teeth; the New York and New Jersey shores are also abutments. Each false tooth on the span is called a *pontic,* which is Latin for bridge unit. When there is no posterior, or rearward, tooth that can serve as a sound abutment, then a removable partial denture is usually the only feasible restoration. In other cases where sound posterior abutments exist, and where not too many teeth are missing, the fixed bridge is the superior restoration.

Sound abutment teeth are crucial to the success of a partial, which can attach to the abutments in any of a variety of ways. The most common attachment is called the clasp, known to most patients as a hook. The circumferential clasp usually has two arms which almost wholly encircle the abutment teeth, thus helping to hold the denture in place. Many other types of clasps and attachments are used, including ingenious precision attachments of great variety and high cost. The special function of each of the many varieties of clasps and attachments are beyond the scope of this book; suffice it to say that the denture is designed, and the attachments selected, with a view to developing the least possible lateral stresses on the abutment teeth, since such stresses tend to weaken the bone support of the teeth. A carefully designed partial will minimize this difficulty, but any type of attachment, no matter how well made, will cause some lateral stresses. For this reason abutment teeth must have sound bone support to begin with if the denture is to succeed for any length of time.

Teeth needed for abutment purposes can often be strengthened by periodontal treatment. This idea of "strengthening" a tooth is much misunderstood. As discussed in the chapter on Disease of the Gums, a tooth is strong only it if is securely held by the jaw, that is, if it has sound bone support. A tooth may be horribly mutilated by caries, but as long as its bone support is sound, it can be restored through regular dental procedures (filling, inlay, or crown) and made to serve as a sound abutment. But a tooth with poor bone support can only be strengthened by periodontal means, if at all. The common notion that a tooth can be strengthened by "capping" (making a crown) is false; a tooth with weak bone support, if crowned, will become a weak tooth with a crown.

Several periodontal procedures have been successfully used to strengthen potential abutment teeth. The weak tooth can be splinted, or permanently attached, to one or more stronger adjacent teeth. This treatment enables all the teeth within the splint to act as a single unit; the strength of the stronger teeth is added to that of the weak tooth to form a sound abutment. Splints are popular, and they usually produce excellent results. But when the bone support is weak, as it is when splints must be used, other periodontal work should be done on a regular basis, as described elsewhere, to help prevent further weakening.

Once the dentist is satisfied as to the soundness of the abutment teeth, and after the periodontal work is completed, then he must give attention to the engineering aspects of the partial. The device must be planned and designed so as to function efficiently and comfortably without generating too much stress on the abutments and without distorting the forces of occlusion. Any shortcoming in either regard would lead to periodontal damage to the abutment teeth. One can get some idea of the destructive forces that may be generated by a partial denture from the experience of the many partial-denture patients who have found that one or more of their abutment teeth have loosened so much that they must be extracted. Careful design and preparation can keep such failures to a minimum.

Another engineering consideration is what is called the *path of insertion*. A partial should go into place in only one way, just as the lid of a well-made box should go on in one way only; this one way is the path of insertion. When a well-made partial is in place it should feel fully seated, but it should never have to be forced or snapped into place. (But some exceptional types of precision attachments *are* designed to snap in.)

Once sound abutments have been provided and the proper path of insertion is established, the final design of the partial should be planned. Often it will be desirable at this stage to prepare the abutment teeth to receive the attachments of the partial. Rest seats are often cut into the abutments; these are shallow, saucer-shaped indentations into which corresponding parts of the partial will fit. Only when all these preparations are completed will the dentist be ready for impressions.

Many variations are possible in the design and construction of partials. There are all-metal cases with baked-in or cemented tooth facings that use no plastic, and there are all-plastic cases which use no metal. The final design, of course, will vary with the requirements of the individual case. Most partials have a metal framework that supplies a very precise fit. Gold was formerly the only metal used for this framework, but today most partial frameworks are cast of a chromiun-cobalt-nickel alloy which in most respects is greatly superior to gold. The modern alloys are lighter and stronger and even more tarnish-resistant than the gold alloys. They are also easier to keep clean. Acrylic plastic is usually used for the pink, gum-like areas of the appliance, called *saddles* or *tissue-bearing areas*. These tissue-bearing areas supply additional stability. They rest firmly against the gum in areas from which teeth have been extracted, or against the hard palate. The false teeth, of porcelain or plastic, are set into the acrylic.

As in so much of dentistry, the key to success with partial dentures is *time,* the time that the dentist is willing to spend with his patient. A partial denture *can* be made in very little time, and many are, by taking a quick impression and "bite" (a hasty jaw registration) and having the laboratory take over from there. The restoration that will result is much less likely to succeed than the partial that is thoughtfully conceived and carefully prepared. Many patients view the partial as a step on the road to full dentures. It has been their experience that abutment teeth keep loosening until they must be extracted, and that more teeth and new clasps then have to be added to the partial. This process continues over the years until so few teeth are left that the full denture is inevitable. But, as we have seen, carefully planned partials for which the mouth has been well prepared need not give such a poor result.

The *Nesbitt* is a unilateral (one-side-of-the-mouth) short-span partial which replaces only one tooth, or occasionally two. A few (very few) authorities consider the Nesbitt an acceptable restoration; most strongly condemn it. Nesbitt appliances usually generate damaging stresses of great magnitude on the abutment teeth; the result is often failure and loss of the abutments. Fixed bridgework is vastly superior to the Nesbitt for replacing one or two teeth.

The Nesbitt is one of Dr. Poorwork's favorite prosthetic devices. It is very easy to make, it costs him only ten to twenty dollars in laboratory fees, and it requires perhaps ten minutes of his valuable chair time. And then there is the prospect of making another Nesbitt in a few years, after the present gadget has loosened an abutment tooth sufficiently to warrant extraction. *For each such device the patient may pay one hundred dollars or more.* In addition to its huge profit per minute of chair time, the Nesbitt has the further advantage that it is much less expensive than fixed bridgework. Thus it enables Dr. Poorwork to maintain his reputation for reasonable fees without compromising his practice of making unreasonable profits.

Good oral hygiene habits are particularly important for wearers of partial dentures. If food residues and film are allowed to accumulate on clasps, which are food traps, the abutment teeth may decay. Some dentists who do not trust their patients to keep their teeth clean make protective crowns for the abutment teeth. The principles of oral hygiene for partial dentures are similar to those described in the chapter Dentures: Hygiene and Hazards.

If a partial denture breaks or becomes damaged in any way, it should be taken at once to the dentist for repair. Attempts to wear a damaged appliance can be dangerous. A partial denture is engineered so as to equalize the stresses bearing on the remaining teeth. Any deformation of the appliance can subject an abutment tooth to greater stress, which in turn may cause bone resorption and loosening of the tooth. A shift of a fraction of a millimeter in the form of the partial can establish destructive forces on several teeth. Any change in the occlusion can cause loss of bone support or contribute to temporomandibular joint disorders, and any change in tissue fit can cause sores, chronic irritations, and even malignancies. It should be obvious that amateur attempts to repair a denture are fraught with danger. Do-it-yourself dentistry is high folly.

20

Fixed Bridgework

The fixed bridge is more costly, more difficult to make, and takes more time than the removable partial denture, but the patient willing to endure these inconveniences will be greatly rewarded by its advantages. When feasible, fixed bridgework is, by far, modern dentistry's best replacement for missing teeth. And although a fixed bridge is not always practicable, it is likely that a high percentage of all people who have removable partial dentures could have been better served with fixed prostheses.

Chief among its advantages are convenience, comfort, efficiency in function, and longevity. The fixed bridge is inserted permanently and stays in; the patient will not be embarrassed by the appliance coming out during a meal or in a social situation. The fixed bridge does not have the unesthetic and often visible extraneous attachments necessary for the partial; there are no lingual or palatal bars or clasps to engage the tongue and interfere with mouth movements. The new partial wearer often has to relearn to speak because of these attachments, while the fixed-bridge patient has no such inconvenience. The fixed bridge feels much like one's own teeth. It does not come out, and it does not have to be removed after every meal for cleaning, as does a partial. The fixed bridge, since it is carefully designed to distribute stresses among the abutment teeth in the safest manner, and because it is stronger than the partial, can be better used for heavy chewing. If properly cared for, furthermore, carefully planned and well-executed fixed bridgework can be expected to give much longer service than a removable denture replacing the same teeth.

But, as we shall see, the construction of a fixed bridge calls for high levels of skill and application from the dentist; partials are easier to do. Fixed bridgework is quite expensive, and does not necessarily return a high profit to the dentist; removable bridgework costs the patient much less and returns a proportionately higher profit to the dentist. These reasons go far to explain why partials are so much more popular than the fixed appliances. Still, the merits of the fixed bridge are such that more and more patients are today being educated to recognize its general superiority.

Though most bridges have abutments at each end of the bridge, one occasionally sees a false tooth that is anchored to one abutment only; in effect the denture has been hung onto the abutment tooth to form a *cantilever bridge*. Such a bridge is theoretically unsound because of the enormous leverage exerted on the abutment; it is as if a bridge that had been built across the Niagara River were attached only to the Canadian shore. Yet cantilever bridges can be used in certain cases when the abutment is reinforced.

A fuller understanding of fixed bridgework may be

gained from a brief outline of the major steps in the construction of a fixed bridge that is to replace one missing tooth. Let us take the lower right first molar, or six-year molar, as an example of the missing tooth.

First the mouth must be studied and the potential abutments analyzed. The preparations of the abutment teeth must allow for considerations of parallelism, occlusion, and esthetics. Once the dentist is satisfied that the bridge can be made successfully, work can begin. The teeth on both sides of the empty space are next prepared to receive full crowns. This involves the removal of sufficient bulk of tooth structure, by grinding the tooth down, to allow for placement of a strong crown. Patients who think that the dentist is taking away too much of the tooth should remember that a considerable amount of grinding is necessary to allow for sufficient bulk of the restorative material, usually veneered gold, as well as to insure that the crowns are parallel to each other (or the finished bridge won't go into place).

Impressions of the abutment teeth are taken only after the grinding has been completed. There are many impression techniques, and many different materials are used. Suffice it to say that any impression technique, to work properly, must be employed with great care, and that any good technique in the hands of a good dentist will deliver an impression from which an exact duplicate of the prepared tooth can be made. It is on this exact duplicate, or die, of the tooth that the crown will be made and fitted. Other impressions are then taken to register the relationships with adjoining teeth and the occlusal, or bite, relationships with the opposing teeth of the other jaw. From all these impressions and registrations an accurate duplicate of the patient's mouth is constructed on which to make the crowns.

At this visit, after the crown preparations are made and the impressions taken, the patient is supplied with a temporary bridge, or temporary crowns, to keep the prepared abutment teeth covered and protected, and to prevent movement of the abutments until the permanent bridge is ready for cementation. Teeth will often move about in the mouth if not stabilized by contact with adjacent or opposing teeth. Once a tooth has been ground down for a crown preparation, it no longer is in contact with adjoining or opposing teeth, and it is prone to shift position in the mouth. Should this happen, the crowns being made will not fit and the teeth will have to be reprepared. The temporary bridge stabilizes the teeth and restores occlusal and proximal contact of the abutment teeth with their neighbors. The temporary bridge also serves to keep the newly ground teeth covered and protected from the irritating action of food and the oral fluids.

One can see that a great deal of work must be accomplished in this visit: Tooth preparations, various impressions, and construction and fitting of a temporary bridge. This is all demanding work that must be meticulously done. Many dentists find it convenient to schedule a visit of several hours to accomplish it all.

At the next visit the temporary bridge is temporarily removed, and the newly made crowns are checked for fit, marginal adaptation, occlusion, and contact with the next tooth. Necessary adjustments are made; occasionally a crown proves unsatisfactory and has to be remade from new impressions. Once the dentist is satisfied that the crowns are correct, then further impressions are taken with the crowns in place over the abutment teeth to register the proper position of each crown relative to the other; from this registration a false tooth will be made and fitted between the abutment crowns, and the whole assembly will be soldered together to form the framework of the bridge. The dentist now puts the temporary bridge back in place and dismisses the patient.

At the next visit the assembled framework, consisting of the metal crowns and the false tooth, soldered together to form one unit, is checked in the mouth for fit. If the fit is satisfactory, another registration is taken, this one for the construction of the plastic or porcelain veneers which will go over the gold for esthetic reasons. On the next visit, which may be the final one, the completed and polished bridge is checked and, if it is satisfactory, can then be cemented permanently into place. The temporary bridge is at last retired.

As is obvious from the above, a fixed bridge can involve many hours of difficult, tedious, highly skilled work—and all to replace one tooth! Neighborhood fees may be between $250 to $350 for a fixed bridge of this size. Contrast this with the one-tooth removable partial denture, the Nesbitt, which takes perhaps five to fifteen minutes to make. It is ironical that at average neighborhood fees a dentist can show as much profit for making a Nesbitt in ten minutes as he can for making a fixed bridge with all the attendant hard work.

The summary given above is of a popular bridge technique. Different techniques include some which telescope some visits and utilize shortcuts that can eliminate others. These techniques often produce excellent results, but sometimes they lead to imperfect bridges; then the entire bridge must be done over, from start to finish. But a dentist who uses such a technique, and who sees something wrong in his work, may be inclined to ignore the imperfection and thereby save himself the inconvenience of backtracking to correct it. The result can only be a bridge that will not serve as well as it should. I have seen such defective bridges in patients' mouths, bridges which were made in factory-style offices where several dentists employed accelerated techniques. Although some of these offices have good reputations, even here poor work does sneak through, very likely because of the high-speed techniques used. But too much is at stake to work so hastily. Most dentists prefer methods much like the one outlined, in which each succeeding step is carefully checked before going ahead to the next step, so that necessary corrections can be made at any time during the procedure.

21

Full Dentures

The mouth with no teeth in it represents the ultimate failure of dentistry and is the most difficult to treat satisfactorily. The best-made denture for the most receptive mouth is but a very poor substitute for the natural dentition. This point is dramatized by a calculation that, even when the best techniques and materials of modern dentistry have been used, the eating efficiency of full dentures is only about twenty per cent that of the healthy natural teeth. The results of relatively primitive attempts at full-denture construction must have been appalling. George Washington suffered from bad teeth all his life; when he finally lost them all the pain of toothache was replaced by the chronic discomfort of his poorly fitting, primitive dentures. Our first President tried several types of dentures; he used false teeth of ivory, bone, metal, and wood, but all were miserable. Perhaps the chronic dental suffering he endured contributed to his compassionate nature. Would he have been less of a great man if he had had the advantages of modern dentistry to relieve his pain?

Full dentures are now made of lightweight, strong materials which can be cast and processed to an extremely precise fit. Acrylic plastic is almost always used for the base, or plate; metals and vinyls have also been used. The teeth themselves are constructed of acrylic or vinyl plastic, or porcelain. Porcelain teeth were once preferred because of their superior resistance to abrasion, but the vastly improved plastics are now highly popular.

The dentist to whom a toothless patient has come should first complete a careful oral examination, including X-rays. This examination may uncover conditions that should be treated promptly. Retained roots, cysts, impacted or unerupted teeth, infections, bone diseases, and tumors are among the conditions which may be present and should be corrected before dentures are made. Occasionally the tissues are in poor condition— puffy, inflamed, not firm. (Recently developed tissue treatments using soft relining materials have proved successful in conditioning tissues that in many cases would previously have required surgery.)

Once the examination is concluded, and the dentist is satisfied that it is all right to proceed, he begins to make a series of impressions and measurements, that must be checked and rechecked at different stages of construction. Measurement is taken of the centric relation and vertical dimension, which essentially are the correct biting relationships of the two jaws consistent with the functional movement of the temporomandibular joint, where the upper and lower jaws meet. These and other relationships must be carefully established, and then verified and reverified. If all this is not done, the dentures may fit the tissues but not the movements of the jaw apparatus. Dentures made to incorrect jaw relationships are especially inefficient, and may cause serious temporomandibular joint malfunction and pain. (See the chapter on Disease of the Gums.)

Not surprisingly, there are differences of opinion as to the precise best way to make the impressions; there are, after all, dozens of impression techniques and materials to choose from. Various compounds, waxes, self-hardening pastes, quick-curing plastics, latex-type compounds, and plasters are available. The choice of material is affected by the structural requirements of the mouth, the condition of the tissues, and the preference of the operator. Preliminary impressions are often taken simply in order to construct a tray to be used to take a corrected, more detailed final impression. In the absence of conclusive proof to the contrary, it seems that satisfactory results can be obtained with almost any accepted impression technique, provided only that the work is done with care.

During the first few visits accurate impressions are taken, models made from these impressions, and jaw relationships established. False teeth are selected as to size, shape, and color, and are tried in the mouth. The initial work on the dentures is not completed until the dentist has settled all the technical problems, and both dentist and patient are satisfied with the appearance.

Now comes the ticklish adjustment period, which is crucial to the patient's ability to learn to use the dentures, and which calls for patience and understanding on the part of the dentist. During the adjustment period the dentist must correct all deficiencies of fit and occlusion. The causes of any sores resulting from the wearing of the denture must be found and corrected. The most common cause of denture sores from a well-made denture is extension of the borders too far into the cheek, lip, tongue, or palate areas. The dentist must exercise great care in making these border adjustments; if a border is cut too short, loss of fit will result, while if it is left too long, tissue sores and irritations will follow. Adjustments should be made cautiously over a period of time; the careful dentist does not go in for massive adjustments and thereby risk a loss of fit in his anxiety to relieve sores and complete the case. The occlusion is checked and rechecked during the adjustment period, which can usually be completed during several visits over two or three weeks, but sometimes takes much longer, perhaps depending upon the patient's ability to learn to handle the dentures. All these procedures take time, that essential commodity which any professional man must be prepared to give if he is to render his best service.

The patient's attitude is crucial to the success of the dentures, and it follows that the dentist must generate a favorable attitude by being particularly sensitive to the patient's emotional state. This is no easy job; it takes an experienced, well-trained, compassionate dentist who is willing to stay with his patient as long as necessary.

The psychology of the successful treatment of denture patients can be quite complex. Often the patient is elderly, with the anxieties usually attendant on old age. Younger patients may feel prematurely old; with them, the false teeth symbolize a milestone in the relentless passing of time. Some patients' anxiety is increased by long histories of pain, discomfort, and inability to eat comfortably because of carious, infected, and periodontally involved teeth. Nearly all denture patients are particularly anxious about their appearance, and many are looking forward hopefully to being able to chew and to eat in comfort again. Such considerations contain obvious and compelling arguments for making every effort to retain some, if not all, of the natural dentition. They also explain why the patient's inability to keep his teeth symbolizes a defeat that may cause him to be profoundly depressed.

It now becomes clear, perhaps, that the treatment of denture patients must give as much attention to the various emotional factors as to the technical aspects of the dentures. The prospective patient must be treated with extreme patience and understanding, but without undue gravity, which might reinforce his gloom. The dentist should listen at length as the patient tells of his troubles with his mouth, and he must be both sympathetic and reassuring. The constructive nature of the work must be stressed, but without promising the moon. If the patient's expectations are too high, a let-down will result, and he may not pass successfully through the adjustment period.

Early in the treatment the patient must be taught exactly what to expect from the completed denture. This education, stressing the constructive aspects, continues with every visit. The following points summarize what the patient must be taught:

1. Dentures are a very poor substitute for natural teeth.
2. They are not held in place firmly, as were the natural teeth, and consequently tend to dislodge with heavy stresses.
3. Successful use will come only after practice and accommodation by the patient, who will learn to handle dentures much as one learns to handle a wooden leg.
4. The adjustment period will be difficult, and may be lengthy and painful.

5. Despite these depressing prospects, however, dentures can be made to look good and to function well enough so that the patient can expect to learn to eat most foods comfortably.

Though the positive aspects must be continually stressed, most patients will do better if they are not led to expect too much. In fact, a somewhat pessimistic outlook is usually desirable; the patient will be delighted if the false teeth prove to be better than expected and the difficulties less than he feared, and he will become self-assured and more quickly skillful in their use. Nevertheless, the attitude of pessimism must be carefully tempered with encouragement, so as to avoid resignation. The successful management of all these considerations rests upon the psychological expertise of the dentist.

A partial denture utilizes the remaining natural teeth in the mouth for attachment and support, but the full denture, having no such source of support, simply rests on the gums. The upper denture rests on the bony ridge of the upper jaw, where the teeth used to be, and it also has the large area of the bony hard palate to rest upon. A lower denture, on the other hand, has much less total area for support; only the horseshoe-shaped ridge of the lower jaw is available. For this reason upper dentures are invariably more successful than lower dentures. The upper stays in place more easily and requires less patience, accommodation, and skill.

The factors which combine to keep a denture in place are many, and they are often subtle. The dentist tries to construct the denture so that the positive factors, that tend to keep it in place, are emphasized to the limit, while the negative factors, that tend to dislodge it, are minimized or eliminated. The most important factor in the retention of the denture is the surface tension of the saliva, which, combined with the action of atmospheric pressure, or suction, causes the tissues and denture base to-cling to each other once they have been put in intimate contact. The more precise the fit, the more intimate the contact between tissue and denture, and the more firmly the denture is retained. The other major factors in the retention of a denture are negative; the trick here is to try to eliminate or cut down on the forces that tend to dislodge it. These negative factors include poor occlusion, poor jaw relationships, overextensions, and certain habits of eating, talking, and so on.

Because of the importance of salivary surface tension, it is desirable to maximize its effect by covering as much tissue as possible with the denture, but without overextending it. An underextended denture does not take full advantage of the possibilities of surface tension. An overextended denture is even worse, because its borders impinge on the movements of the cheeks, lips, and tongue, causing irritations and sore spots. In addition, these muscular movements will repeatedly dislodge such a denture. The denture with proper extensions is largely unaffected by the average range of muscular movements, but any denture will be dislodged by extreme movements. It follows that an important function of the adjustment period is the repatterning of the patient's muscular habits so as to avoid extreme movements. Many habitual patterns of chewing, drinking, speaking, smoking, and singing may have to be modified to accommodate the new dentures. If the denture is to be successful, it is up to the dentist to help the patient make the necessary accommodations.

The bootleg dentist is an unlicensed practitioner, usually a laboratory technician, who will illicitly take impressions and deliver dentures to a patient who has sought out his services because of the lower fee involved. In view of the ramifications and complexities of denture work it is obvious how dangerous it is to try to save money on dentures by using a bootleg dentist, who has absolutely no training outside of laboratory procedures, and who knows nothing about anatomical considerations, jaw relationships, occlusion, or denture-induced lesions. The bootleg dentist will merrily make a denture over tissue in bad condition, over retained roots, infected jaws, even over tumors. After all, he is not trained to diagnose or treat such conditions. A denture placed over loose, unhealthy tissue can lead to very serious consequences, malignancies for example. Similarly, poorly made dentures can be sources of chronic irritation leading to painful lesions and, occasionally, to malignancies. Temporomandibular joint malfunction with attendant pain and headache; dentures that do not stay in place, can't be used for chewing, look poorly—these can be still other consequences of bootleg dentistry. One may ask if the bootleg dentist, with no training, is any worse than Dr. Poorwork, who will not take the time to utilize his training. The bootleg dentist is much worse. At least Dr. Poorwork can recognize sick tissues and interpret X-rays, and he knows how to treat lesions before they become malignant.

In the past a patient about to have his remaining teeth extracted, usually because of periodontal disease, had to endure the inconvenience of doing without teeth for four to six weeks or longer while the gums healed enough so that impressions could be taken and the dentures made. Today the technique of the *immediate denture* has been developed to a point such that the false teeth are now inserted in the mouth immediately following the final extractions. Healing of the sockets of the extracted teeth takes place underneath the immediate denture, which acts somewhat as a dressing and actually eases the discomfort of healing. The immediate denture cannot start off with the precision of fit of the final denture, and as the gums heal, the tissues change, further altering the fit. For this reason new impressions are taken after the healing period; the immediate denture is then rebased to conform precisely to the healed tissues. At this point corrections in occlusion and jaw relationships can also be made. The principle of immediate replacement is not confined to full denture work, but can also be used for both removable and fixed partial prostheses.

Dentures, which under normal conditions do not change in form, are made to fit precisely against tissues which, over periods of time, *do* normally change in form. Just as a person's outward physical appearance changes, so the hard palate, the bony ridges of the upper and lower jaws, the muscles, and the soft tissues of the mouth undergo changes. Inevitably, therefore, a denture which at first fits perfectly against these tissues will gradually lose closeness of fit. Furthermore, an ill-fitting denture will accelerate tissue change by causing irritation, which results in sore and swollen tissues and bone resorption; thus a vicious circle may be set up. Fortunately the reestablishment of a close fit is, as a rule, a relatively simple procedure that is accomplished by relining or rebasing the denture. In effect, that part of the denture which fits against the tissues is remade, while the rest of the denture and its relationships remain undisturbed. This simple and relatively inexpensive work is accomplished through new impressions, some fairly easy laboratory work, and then a small adjustment period. If a denture shows any signs of losing its fit or stability in the mouth, a rebase should be done before any considerable damage to the tissue results. It is partly for this reason that people with dentures should go for regular dental check-ups; periodic examinations of the oral tissues are also advisable.

Dentures are made of plastics and porcelains and metals, and these materials are eminently breakable. Furthermore, any change in a denture, no matter how apparently insignificant, may profoundly change its function and support. If a denture breaks or becomes damaged, no matter how slightly, it should be taken to the dentist at once for repair. Attempts to wear a damaged appliance of any kind can prove very injurious, as by causing a change in tissue fit, with resulting sores and chronic irritations and worse. It should be obvious that do-it-yourself attempts to repair a denture are dangerous.

Spare dentures are considered by many patients to be a convenience well worth the added expense. The second denture can be worn if the primary denture has to be repaired or rebased; in such cases the patient is spared the inconvenience of having to go without teeth while laboratory work is being done on the primary denture. But, except in emergencies, the owner of a second denture should never wear it, since it is not an exact duplicate of the first and the patient should adjust and accommodate himself to wearing one denture only.

For some patients, relative success comes more easily than for others. Anatomically, some patients are much better suited to dentures than others. Patients with large, broad, bony ridges on the jaws have more area for support of the dentures than patients with tiny, resorbed ridges. Patients with eccentric jaw relations, or with too large or too small a vertical dimension, can be expected to have trouble. People with particularly heavy or particularly thin saliva, other factors being equal, have more difficulty than patients with a normal quality and flow of saliva. Yet patients with tiny ridges, poor saliva, grotesque jaw relationships, and unfavorable vertical dimension have been known to get along fine with their dentures, while other patients with large, bony ridges, normal saliva, and ideal jaw relations have sometimes not been able to use dentures at all. These observations strongly suggest that the most important consideration, assuming the best possible fit, is the psychological factor.

Most poorly made dentures are the result of too little time spent by the dentist in planning and executing his work and in preparation of the patient's mouth. Of course, our friend Dr. Poorwork *should* be very skillful with dentures, since he has occasion to make so many of them. Unfortunately, he rarely has the time to do the job well.

The public has been conditioned to accept a high fee for denture service and a relatively low fee for fillings and periodontal work, but the reverse would make more sense. Though the cost of materials in a denture is but a few dollars, fees for new dentures have always been high. Today's quality laboratory fee for full dentures may range from fifty to ninety dollars; this is paid by the dentist. An average neighborhood dentist's fee for full dentures, upper and lower, might be between three and five hundred dollars. Since the average practitioner does not spend much time with his patient, a close computation could only prove that dentures are a most lucrative field for the typical dentist. It is ironic that the end product of neglect and poor dentistry should be so profitable. The construction of full dentures has always been a lucrative field, and one might well wonder why this should be. An old-time dentist whom I respect once told me that it was his belief that high fees were originally established for denture service because the denture represented the last opportunity the dentist had to make money from the patient, and the most had to be made of it. If this is so, and it may well be so, it gives an uncomfortable insight into the operation of economic motivation in the healing arts. It is time, and more than time, that the professions took a fresh look at their aims and ideals.

22

Dentures:
Hygiene and Hazards

All false teeth, and especially removable partial and full dentures, have their own special hygiene requirements and recurrent problems. For almost every problem there are a number of proprietary products that offer an easy solution. But though denture wearers who use such products do not seem to get more comfortable over the years, the proprietors, like Dr. Poorwork himself, have been growing steadily richer off their victims' discomfort. Nearly all the commercial products in this field are worthless, if not actually harmful.

Most denture-cleaning solutions and "soak-overnight" preparations are ineffectual; most denture-cleaning pastes are so abrasive that, if frequently used over a period of time, they may damage the denture; denture adhesive powders should almost never be used, because they are unsanitary, they harbor foodstuffs,

239

they generate odors, they cause inflammation of tissues, and they may mislead the user into putting up with an ill-fitting denture that can produce very serious damage to his mouth, even malignancies. Relining materials to be applied at home, though well advertised, should *never* be used. Relines that are installed without proper supervision change the occlusion and the distance between the upper and lower jaws when the teeth are in contact, and thus can produce serious temporomandibular joint malfunction, chronic headache and earache, and denture sores. (See chapter on Disease of the Gums.)

Preparations advertised as denture pain-killers lend themselves to misuse in a particularly insidious fashion. These products usually contain an anesthetic agent such as benzocaine, which dulls the pain of a denture sore but does nothing to relieve its cause. To repair or refit a denture at home, and then to doctor the resulting sores with a pain-killer, can have the most serious consequences. A denture wearer should *never* attempt to repair or adjust a denture himself, and should *never* try to tolerate pain, swelling, or a poorly fitting denture. These can be danger signs, and in almost all cases can easily be corrected by the dentist before any serious damage occurs. A chronic denture sore that is merely tolerated or treated with a pain-killer instead of being shown to a dentist is very dangerous and can become malignant.

Dentures must be kept scrupulously clean, or tissue irritations can result. The time to clean dentures is after eating. The best way to clean them is with a brush. A toothbrush can be used, although there are some specially designed brushes that do an excellent job. Toothpaste should not be used; it is too abrasive. Probably the best cleaning agent is a very mild soap, and only occasionally something a little more abrasive, such as a commercial denture cleaner (but not the soak type) can be used. It is wise to stand over a sink *filled* with water when scrubbing a removable denture. Soapy dentures can be very slippery, and are less likely to break if they drop into a water-filled sink than if they fall on a hard floor.

Should dentures be taken out of the mouth at night? In the absence of any instructions from the dentist, who may have a specific reason for wanting the dentures in or out at night, it is usually best for the patient to do what is most comfortable. Wear the dentures if it is comfortable to do so; if not, they should be soaked overnight in *water only*. But this instruction is controversial: Some good dentists recommend that dentures be removed every night, whether or not it is comfortable to keep them in.

There is a relatively new commercial device that may help to clean dentures without damaging them, but it is still too early to judge whether it is likely to damage the plastic of the dentures. The device creates supersonic currents in a water bath that contains a cleaning solution, usually a detergent. This little machine does a good job of cleaning a stubbornly dirty denture. But is it safe? Time will tell.

PART 5

INSURING CARE
AND QUALITY

23

Fees:
At the Root of Evil

Fees are an inescapable part of the framework of private practice, since they are the means by which the dentist is paid for his work. With the recent advent of various types of insurance plans, prepayment plans, and government programs such as Medicaid, some of the fee relationship is being reoriented from doctor-patient to doctor-institution. This is solving some old problems and generating some new ones. But the great majority of fees are still paid by the patient, out of his own pocket.

Fees are the biggest source of frustration for most dentists and the biggest source of misunderstanding by patients. To the conscientious dentist, a patient represents a professional challenge: Here is a person with problems of oral health to be solved. The dentist would like to establish a diagnosis and follow through with the correct treatment. Often, however, he finds that the fee stands between him and the necessary and proper treatment. Sometimes the needed treatment may be out of the patient's reach. Other times he can afford the treatment, but doesn't believe it's worth the price, perhaps despite the best educational efforts of the dentist. Too often, the dentist may not bother to prescribe the best possible course of action, because he believes the patient will never accept costly restorative work. In such cases many dentists prescribe an inferior and less expensive solution in the hopes of achieving acceptance. One result of this approach is that the patient is never given the opportunity to choose between a superior restoration and one which cannot be expected to serve him so well.

Much of the dentist's problem derives from the patient's ignorance. The typical patient believes, because the dentists have allowed him to believe, that there is a fixed cost attached to each dental operation. It is the set fee that has led the patient to this mistaken idea. The set fee, or unit-fee system, has created all kinds of mischief for the dental profession. Yet the unit fee—so-and-so much for a filling, so much for a cleaning, so much for a crown, and so on—is used by almost every practitioner in the country. Unit fees are even specified in the published fee schedules for various dental insurance programs, including Medicaid.

But allowing a set fee for a filling, just for example, is much like having a fixed fee for mowing a lawn. Lawns come in many sizes; it would be absurd to charge the same amount for mowing the biggest and the smallest of lawns. Yet dentistry has, by and large, been tied down to just such an absurd notion throughout its history. Furthermore, the set fee makes no allowance for differences in approach, dedication, and quality of work. To pay the same fee to a good dentist for a large and difficult filling which might have taken an hour to do as one would pay to Dr. Poorwork for his five-minute mishandling of the same job is certainly irrational. Yet this is just what Medicaid and various insurance plans do, and this is just what many patients, seeking out a dentist, expect to do. ("After all," the patient reasons, "A filling is a filling; why should I pay more?") Ridiculous though this situation is, it is likely to continue until the public comes to understand more about the real nature of dental costs and fees.

The dentist does not sell fillings or gold or silver or porcelain or hardware. He has spent many years going to school and training himself for his job. When he is at last ready to offer his services to the public, he has one item and one item only to sell, and that is his *time*. The reason his time is valuable is that his long, specialized training has made it so. Those who need dental work, and therefore purchase a little or a lot of the dentist's time, must pay him what he asks for himself in addition to their proportionate share of his fixed overhead. The dentist sets a monetary value on his time by comparing how much time he has available to sell with the annual income he hopes to achieve. Thus fees per unit of time depend on three factors: (1) the cost of the dentist's overhead per unit of time; (2) how much annual income the dentist plans to earn with his time; and (3) how much time he has to sell.

The first factor the dentist considers is the amount of time he has available to sell. This means *chair time,* the amount of time actually spent working on the patient, the amount of actual *productive* working time. In an average eight-hour day at the office the dentist may find that his productive chair time is six hours or less, the rest of the time being taken up by laboratory work, the telephone, the planning of treatment, talking to patients or their parents or other relatives, and so on. If we now include time-wasters such as missed appointments, sickness of patients or doctor, late-coming patients, the growing volume of insurance and government forms to fill out, and other paper work, we find that six productive chair-hours per day is a generous estimate. Calculating on a four-and-a-half day week, which is long enough in view of the brutal physical demands on the conscientious dentist, and allowing for vacations and "slow periods," such as July, August, and December, when the dentist may not be fully scheduled, and excluding time taken with hospital staff assignments, voluntary work, and dental meetings, our hypothetical dentist may average twelve to thirteen hundred hours of chair time a year.

Productive chair time must not be confused with actual working time, which is much greater. A dentist with twenty-eight hours of productive chair time in a week is not working a twenty-eight hour week; it is more likely, when all his working hours are considered, that he is putting in forty hours. The analogy with teaching is instructive. A public-school teacher spends fewer than twelve hundred hours yearly in the classroom, but presumably spends much additional time preparing lessons, reading papers, conferring with parents, and so forth. In the course of a full year a college professor may spend fewer than four hundred hours in the classroom, but may need up to four times as many hours for preparation, research, and writing. The compensation of the teacher and the professor takes the form of an annual salary that bears little or no relation to the number of hours in the classroom. Unlike the teacher or professor, however, the dentist gets paid only for his *actual productive time*. In his case, this means chair time. The system of payment for the wage earner differs in that he is generally paid in relation to time at the job, whether it is productive work time or not.

Calculating overhead is simpler. The dentist merely adds up his total office expense over a year's time and compares it with his effective chair time. In the New York City area, ten dollars per patient-hour is a decidedly *low* estimate for hourly (chair-hourly, that is) overhead, so let us use that conservative figure. The overhead is, of course, all-inclusive; it takes in equipment depreciation, rent, assistants' salaries, laboratory charges, supplies, utilities, cleaning, and so forth. Let us for the moment, then, consider that the cost of all this comes to only ten dollars per chair-hour, or $12,000 annually for the 1,200 chair-hours.

In the final phase of his computation the dentist must address himself to the ticklish notion of his own worth, or how much he deserves to make in annual income. Having decided on this figure, he divides it by the number of hours that represent his annual chair time (1,200) and adds to this quotient his computed hourly overhead, or $10. The result is the fees he must average per chair-hour to attain his desired annual income. Let us suppose for a moment that the aimed-for annual income is $12,000. Dividing this by 1,200 (available chair-hours), we get $10 per hour; adding to this $10 (hourly overhead), we get $20. This, then, represents the sum of the fees this dentist must average per hour if he is to achieve his goal of $12,000 income. This is not a heady sum if one has to cope with the cost of living in New York, Denver, or Chicago and must at the same time try to maintain something like a "doctor's living standard." If, instead of $12,000, this dentist decided to earn $24,000 a year, he would have to average $30 per chair-hour in fees. The first $10 of this would cover his overhead, and the balance of $20 would be "profit." In fact, most good dentists today consider their time to be worth $30 per chair-hour.

Assuming the $12,000 annual-income figure, a patient who misses an appointment scheduled for a full hour cost the dentist $20. Of this, $10 is in earnings and the other $10 is in what it costs to keep the office running for that hour. If a dentist works on a filling for an hour and charges only $10, he has earned nothing; all the money must go for overhead. If he charges $12 for an hour, he has worked at the rate of $2 for that chair-hour; at that rate he would earn an annual income of only $2,400. The dentist working on an income goal of $12,000 must accustom his patients to paying a fee of $20 for an hour's visit, of $10 for a half-hour. This must be the *real* basis for the dentist's fee scale.

But very few dentists have been willing to charge on an hourly basis. Traditionally it hasn't been done that way, perhaps from fear that the patient could never understand it. A patient who earns five dollars an hour at his job may conclude that twenty dollars an hour is an enormous salary for a man to make, never considering the doctor's overhead or the difference between chair time and working time, which, if included in the calculations, would bring the dentist's actual hourly wage very near to his own five dollars an hour. To avert such misunderstandings, and because of tradition, most dentists have attempted to translate this hourly fee into unit-work fees. This is done, though not too successfully, by trying to calculate the average time a certain type of procedure takes to accomplish, and charging accordingly. A procedure usually taking an hour costs twenty dollars; the fee for a half-hour procedure is ten dollars. This is the true rationale behind dental fees, though it is not understood at all by most dental patients nor, apparently, by the great majority of insurance-plan administrators, who expect fees to be calculated on a unit-fee basis—so much for a filling, and so on.

In practice, the attempt to break down the necessary hourly fee into work units leads to an unwieldy and irrational structure, which the dentist hopes will average out over the year, so that he will be able to earn his desired income. The contradictions of the unit-fee system lead to serious inequities and abuse. In fact it is the unit-fee system, more than any other factor, which promotes Poorwork-style dentistry.

Tradition and competition for patients usually cause the dentist setting up a new practice to adopt the prevailing local scale of fees for everyday work. He soon finds that some fillings take much more time than others, and decides he cannot afford to charge the same for all fillings. Again following in the footsteps of other dentists, he begins to charge for "surfaces" rather than fillings. A single, large filling in one tooth may involve several surfaces of the tooth; he charges for each surface. The patient, knowing that the dentist charges the prevailing neighborhood fee of five dollars for a filling, may want to know why the filling in one tooth cost fifteen dollars. The dentist explains that there were "three fillings in that tooth." By this he means that the single filling extended over three surfaces. This misleading explanation is an effort to justify the larger fee the dentist needs for a filling that takes much more time than the average filling.

Cavities involving the pulp, which require careful, time-consuming work, such as pulp-capping or pulpotomy, are more difficult to explain to the patient who has never heard of such procedures. But the same patient may have heard of a "tooth treatment," and he may be quite willing to accept that as justification for an additional fee. By now one can begin to see what linguistic contortions the dentist must go through in order to justify a fee that will enable him to make a living.

The word *cleaning* has an even less precise meaning than *filling*. Ideally, when a cleaning has been completed there should be no calculus, plaque, or food debris left in the mouth, which should indeed be clean. But to accomplish this result for most patients a careful periodontal scaling or curettage must be completed; this may take many visits. A "cleaning" might, perhaps, be taken to mean the polishing of the teeth after all the necessary dental work, including periodontal work, has been completed. But for many people a "cleaning" is a perfunctory, partial removal of some calculus, plus a polishing. This is why the good dentist may find it difficult to get a typical patient, accustomed to paying perhaps five dollars for a "cleaning," to accept essential periodontal work. Some dentists have used the term *gum treatments* to justify an adequate unit fee for periodontal work, but this term also lends itself to abuse.

It is easy to derive a unit fee for X-rays. "So much for each X-ray" is easy and obvious, but also ridiculous, since it seems to imply that the material costs and the work involved in each individual X-ray has much of a bearing on the fee. The cost of an X-ray film is about five cents. The cost of the X-ray machine may be a thousand dollars. But the dentist is not trying to pay for the film and amortize the cost of the X-ray machine through his fees for X-rays. The machine and film are part of his essential diagnostic facilities, and their cost is part of his overhead. The fee for an X-ray examination should reflect the service performed by the dentist in his skilled interpretation of the patient's condition, using the X-rays as a diagnostic aid. The patient is not buying a five-cent X-ray film or the use of a thousand-dollar machine; he is buying the diagnostic skill and *time* of the dentist. There is no reason why five X-rays should cost five times as much as one X-ray; the dentist's time is what counts.

Fees for extractions hardly need concern us here. In the good, general practice, the extraction is a rare occurrence. Suffice it to say here that the average extraction can be done in a very few minutes. Specialists' fees are something else; operations usually performed by the specialist on impacted teeth, and so forth, may vary in fee scale.

Fees for fixed and removable bridgework, crowns, jackets, and dentures are generally high, though they vary according to the type of restoration. Such fees are exceptional in that they do not generally reflect a charge for the dentist's time. This is most notably true in the case of full dentures and removable bridgework. The reason usually given to justify this higher rate of return is that prosthetic restorations, or false teeth, carry with them a high degree of responsibility to the patient. This is nonsense; the dentist assumes no less responsibility for any of the work he performs.

The real reason for the high fees for prosthetic dentistry is simply that the patient is willing to accept high fees for such work. Somehow the typical patient has come to believe that false teeth, "caps," "plates," and so on, are worth a lot of money; the dentist capitalizes on the patient's mistake by taking a higher fee, per hour of his time, without risking a serious complaint from the patient. This error on the part of the public probably dates from the days when dentures were carved from wood, ivory, or porcelain, or cast or hand-wrought in metal. To get such dentures to fit was a rare accomplishment: George Washington's troubles with his many sets of dentures are notorious. In his day it took a great amount of time, effort, and skill to make false teeth, and the fees were accordingly high. But with today's efficient impression materials, and with the plastics and porcelains and metal-casting techniques now available, full dentures and removable bridgework can be made in relatively little time and relatively cheaply. Of course, the conscientious dentist must take as much time as necessary for the preparatory work, and after the prosthesis is made he spends however much time is needed for adjustments. But full dentures and partial bridgework nevertheless command fees well in excess of what the dentist would charge on an hourly fee basis. The possibilities for abuse in this situation are obvious: An unscrupulous dentist may tend to prescribe such restorations in place of superior restorations that allow him less profit. This does not hold true for inlays, fixed bridges, or crowns. Such fixed restorations take up more of the dentist's time than do removable appliances, and the fees charged for them are more nearly in line with the dentist's projected hourly fee.

I have mentioned that the unit-fee system is a prime cause for the existence of Poorwork dentistry. An examination of the effects of the system will show why. In a free economic system based on the profit motive it is natural for a man to analyze his work to see if he can make more money from it. The factors that control a dentist's income are his available chair time, his overhead per unit of chair time, and his fees per unit of chair time. To increase his income, the dentist must increase his available chair time, increase his fees per unit of time, or decrease his overhead per unit of time. Most dentists find it impossible to decrease overhead. In the matter of chair time, most dentists, except those who are just getting established, might be unwilling to increase their working hours; the work is difficult and fatiguing. But many a dentist may find it possible to organize his working time more efficiently, so as to allow more chair time per day without increasing working time. This can be done by having an assistant who performs many of the time-consuming, away-from-the-chair tasks, such as paper work, billing, minor laboratory procedures (X-ray development, and so on), appointment-making, etc. The assistant can also be delegated to do most of the talking to patients and parents, in effect taking over the public relations end of the practice. Most practice-management manuals deal at length with methods of increasing the money-efficiency of the dentist's office time. Still, there is a limit to the amount of chair time that can be squeezed out of one day.

The most obvious way to raise income is to increase the basic hourly fee. In the previous example, the dentist worked on a base fee of $20 per hour, and he earned $12,000 yearly. If he increased his hourly fee to $25, his income would rise to $18,000 per year. But an increase in fees, if openly presented, will usually meet with resistance.

No such resistance is encountered, however, if the dentist, taking his first firm step toward Poorworkism, boosts his hourly fee in a concealed manner. This is how it works: The patient is accustomed to accepting a given fee for a unit of work; thus a filling, or surface, is five dollars, a two-surface filling is ten dollars, and so forth. Let us say that the two-surface filling takes a half hour of chair time, which would be consistent with the dentist's basic twenty-dollar-per-chair-hour fee. Having learned that he cannot safely raise the unit fee, the dentist alters the other factor, the chair time per work unit. He simply cuts the working time for a two-surface filling, for instance, to twenty minutes, and instead of being able to do only two such jobs an hour, he can now do three. Thus, by a little sleight of hand, he has raised his effective hourly fee to thirty dollars. It is true that a half-hour job cannot be done properly in twenty minutes, but faced with the pressures of the cost of living, kids in school, a luxury-loving wife ("Dr. Z. and his wife go to Puerto Rico every year; why can't we?"), the dentist has decided that, since the patient will never know the difference, and all the other neighborhood dentists do the same thing anyway, and a happy wife is more important than professional integrity, and nobody appreciates a martyr anyhow, he, too, will do the twenty-minute job.

And so another Poorwork is born. A few years later this dentist has picked up more of the corner-cutting tricks. The twenty-minute filling now takes only ten minutes. Where previously he would extend each surface properly, now he merely makes two or three tiny pits on a tooth surface, and charges for two or three surfaces. If the patient complains, the dentist holds up a mirror so that he or she can count them. The patient never knows that this is very bad dentistry, or that the pitted surface is odds-on to decay again. The new Dr. Poorwork takes to routinely doing temporary fillings, partly for the sedative effect against the pain caused by the remaining decay which he didn't take the time to remove, and partly in order to charge an additional fee for the temporary filling. The patient, being used to paying for units of work, accepts the extra charge without complaint. Useless gentian violet "gum treatments" replace time-consuming periodontal scaling; quick-and-easy extractions take the place of difficult and intricate restorative procedures; cheap, removable bridgework is installed when fixed bridgework is needed. In short, all the sins of bad dentistry discussed at length in this book are gradually incorporated into the practice of this new Dr. Poorwork, and all in the interest of saving time. The single, common characteristic of bad dentistry is that all its work *takes much less time* to accomplish than the analogous procedures of good dentistry. Shoddy dentistry does not reflect poor training, or imcompetence, or lack of continuing education, but only the dentist's observation that *bad work takes less time and therefore enables him to make more money through the unit-fee system.*

When a person buys an everyday, necessary item in a store, his estimate of its worth takes into account the material used in its manufacture. By analogy, the public has come to think that the reason a gold filling costs more than a silver filling is that gold costs more than silver. Actually, the reason the gold filling is more expensive is that it is more difficult to make, takes much more time, and usually involves a laboratory fee. The extra materials cost, of perhaps two dollars, is insignificant. Similarly, a patient may believe that a removable appliance replacing seven teeth is worth more than a fixed appliance replacing two teeth, when in fact the fixed appliance takes much more time, involves a higher laboratory fee, and requires a much higher fee than the larger removable appliance. Patients are ready and willing to pay twice as much for the extraction of four teeth in one area of the mouth as they would expect to pay for the extraction of only two; yet the time and effort involved for the dentist are very nearly the same. In the case of the restorations the patient believes are done mainly by the laboratory, he may think the laboratory charge is the most significant part of his fee. And patients have been known to pay an enormous premium for dentures which use false teeth made abroad in the mistaken belief that these false teeth are very superior and much more costly to the dentist. I call the practice of paying for items and materials, instead of for services, "hardware-store dentistry."

In the face of the contrasting economic possibilities of different types of dental work, some practitioners are tempted to prescribe work that returns them the most money per chair-hour. The wary consumer may be interested to learn the degree of profit represented by various forms of work, so that he may consider to what extent the economic factor may have intruded upon the diagnosis and prescription for his case. In the following discussion I will use the unit-fee scale allowed by New York State Medicaid in 1968 as a basis for estimating the profit potential for vaious dental procedures. This scale may not be entirely representative of fees charged by neighborhood dentists, but it is generally close enough for our purposes. While considering what follows, the reader should keep in mind: (1) That it is the unit-fee-for-unit-work system that allows inconsistencies in potential profit to the dentist; and (2) that in each case where a unit fee is applicable, the less time the dentist spends on the procedure, the more profitable it will be to him and (obviously) the more quickly he will be ready for another patient and another fee.

The silver amalgam filling, probably the most common procedure of all, is also one of the least remunerative for good dentists. The Medicaid scale allows five dollars per surface, up to three surfaces per tooth. A carefully done two-surface filling may take fifteen minutes to an hour or, on the average, a half-hour of chair time. At this rate the Medicaid scale would pay the dentist $20 per hour of chair time, giving him an annual income of $12,000. But a fast-moving Dr. Poorwork can complete his conception of a two-surface amalgam filling in five to ten minutes; thus he will receive for his shoddy, substandard work some three to six times as much as the careful dentist. This illustration, which concerns the commonest of all dental procedures, is sufficient commentary on how the economic motive, working hand-in-glove with the unit-fee scale of Medicaid, can adversely affect the quality of dental work.

Much the same applies to other types of common fillings, particularly the so-called porcelain fillings for front teeth, where silver is esthetically unsuitable. Medicaid allows seven dollars for a silicate anterior filling, with a maximum of eighteen dollars per tooth. These prices bring such fillings in line with silver fillings as far as the dentist's profit is concerned.

Crowns, jackets, and fixed bridgework represent low-income chair time for very difficult work. The New York Medicaid fee scale, which is very low for this type of work, allows $200 for a common three-unit bridge which replaces one missing tooth, and which utilizes veneer crowns on each of the two abutment teeth. This may represent about six difficult hours of chair time. After the dentist pays the laboratory fees, the balance leaves him just a little more than he gets on an hourly basis for routine amalgam fillings. Of course, all kinds of horrendous short-cuts *can* be employed which might reduce working time down to perhaps an hour. These short-cuts result in a terrible piece of work, but increase the profit considerably.

Routine root canal work is more profitable. Medicaid allows a fee of fifty dollars for a simple root canal job. Although the required chair time varies considerably, depending on the case, *on the average* the good dentist can complete a careful root canal filling in three or four visits, with total chair time running to about one and one-half hours. Of course a shoddy job can be completed in less time. Though it has much less chance of succeeding, it is rewarded even more handsomely, per chair-hour by the fixed-fee scale.

Removable false teeth bring the dentist his highest profit. The Medicaid fee scale, low by many dentist's standards, still allows a good return per chair-hour for the dentist for both full and partial denture work, partials being the more lucrative and less time-consuming. Not counting extra fees allowable for extractions, the Medicaid rate for one full denture is $150, which may be less than the usual dentist's fee, but is still high enough to provide a good profit. For an average partial denture Medicaid allows nearly $200 for perhaps one hour's relatively easy work. Dr. Poorwork takes still less time, because he does not bother to prepare the abutment teeth properly. Fees for full and partial removable prostheses have always been high, and have always given the dentist a high rate of return. Quick extractions and hastily made partials have long been a Poorwork trademark. His favorite partial is often the Nesbitt bridge, which replaces one tooth with a removable appliance, and is a generally condemned procedure. To the credit of Medicaid, it evidently will not pay for a Nesbitt.

The New York Medicaid unit-fee scale reflects the dogma of the American Dental Association that there is little or no qualitative difference between dentists, and that all do satisfactory work. But I hope some of the absurdities of a fixed fee scale a la Medicaid have been made clear by the above discussion. The fixed fee rewards speed, and speed is the death of good dentistry. In other words, Medicaid pays much more per hour for shoddy dentistry than it does for good dentistry, which is better for the patient and, in the long run, much cheaper for the state. Here, in a nutshell, is the major paradox for the fixed-fee scale.

In order to avoid misunderstandings, most good dentists invite a full discussion of fees before starting treatment of any new patient. Should the dentist not bring up the subject, the patient most certainly should. Of course, the dentist cannot quote a fee before he has conducted his examination, except that he can, and should, quote a fee for the examination beforehand. As soon as the examination has been completed and treatment plan established, the dentist should, as a rule, be prepared to quote a fee. But sometimes the diagnosis leaves some questions that can be answered only in the course of treatment. In such cases it may be impossible for the dentist to quote a firm fee, though he should nevertheless try to give the patient the clearest possible idea of the fees which may be involved. In the case of specialists, the patient would be well advised to ask about fees before making an appointment.

It is obvious that the fee structure of dentistry needs to be reformed. The unit-fee system, with its built-in incentives for bad dentistry, should be modified or replaced, perhaps by a system based on a time-experience-knowledge factor. The ADA has gone on record with the opinion that fees should be based on knowledge, skill, experience, effort, and responsibility. According to the ADA, it is these factors which provide the basis for the reward of fees. But this ignores the fact that it is not the mere *possession* of knowledge and skill which is important; it is their *use* that matters. Dr. Poorwork has been trained to do good dentistry, and he has shown his ability on school and licensing examinations. But Poorwork does not take the time to use his knowledge and skill, and this is what is important to the patient. The level of dentistry could be almost uniformly high if all dentists took the time to do the best work of which they are capable. But not all dentists do. I suggest that whether the dentist does or does not take the time to do his job properly should be the most significant criterion for establishing his fees.

There should not be great differentials in the hourly reward for different procedures, because excessive differentials provide incentives for the more profitable procedures without regard to the needs of the patient. If all procedures paid a similar rate per chair-hour, with some modest variations for difficulty, all dentists would be more likely to base their plan of treatment on what was best for the patient, since there would be no substantial monetary advantage in any alternative type of treatment.

Except in the specialties, therefore, I would discount the first two of the ADA's published criteria, knowledge and skill, as meaningful bases for differentiation of fees as between different procedures. The ADA's third criterion, effort, is the really significant factor. Effort, translated into time, makes knowledge and skill meaningful; without effort, knowledge and skill are worthless. The ADA's fourth criterion, "Responsibility: effect of error and correction of error," leaves much to be desired. There should be no difference in the degree of responsibility for different dental procedures; the dentist should be completely responsible for all phases of his work. As to error and its correction, the dentist must make every effort to insure that *all* his work is free of error. If his work fails after he has made such an effort, he takes appropriate measures at an additional fee; this is the usual practice. Error and its correction should not be a factor for increasing the initial fee.

Nevertheless, this consideration is often used (and abused) to justify a high initial fee. Here is an example. Some high-fee dentists emphasize rehabilitation procedures as a panacea to patients with problems. "We'll cap all your teeth and you'll never have trouble again" is the pitch. But too often ill-conceived rehabilitations, although done at enormous fees, fail miserably after several years, and the patient is left with few, if any, functional teeth. Where is the remedy for this patient? What relevance have the ADA criteria for this patient, particularly the criterion, "Responsibility: effect of error and correction of error"?

It will not be easy to change the basis for fees. A movement toward a time-based fee structure will be bitterly resisted by the Poorworks. If they converted their work and fee schedules to a time basis, their present methods would be exposed; not only would they have to reform their methods, but they would have to be content with much less income. If they tried to maintain present income levels under a time-based fee system, they would have to present a very high per-time fee to the patient; this would put the lie to the pretense that their fees were reasonable, and would not be likely to be accepted by their patients.

Then there will be the ticklish problem of finding a way to establish equitable time-based fee levels for good dentistry. I believe that the solution will be found most readily through a program designed to teach the patient the facts he needs to know about dentistry and fees. Fees should be negotiated directly with the patient in the light of his full and open knowledge as to what he will be getting, i.e., what dentistry is all about. The knowledgeable patient will not balk at reasonable time-unit fee levels when he understands the nature of the Poorwork alternative.

Implementation of such a scheme would have its hazards. If, for example, the dentist is to get paid on the basis of time, it is possible that incentives to complete work in a reasonable time will be lacking and a tendency to goof off will develop. The unit-fee incentive to produce more work in less time may be replaced by an indifferent attitude expressed in the words, "I'm being paid as much anyhow; why should I knock myself out?" There is no doubt that this hazard exists. The best protection against it would be the competition and professional alertness of a well-run, idealistic group practice. The interested group would not be likely to tolerate the lack of dedication and the lassitude of an indifferent member. The self-discipline of the group would break down only in the case of collusion among all the members of the group. Such collusion would be unlikely to occur, but if it did the group's shortcomings would quickly become obvious to the informed patients, who would not permit it to continue. (These patients would become informed through programs of patient-education). In any case, it seems that the possible problem of laziness must be minute compared to the existing problems of poor quality under the unit-fee system.

The subject of quality raises the question, What place will Dr. Poorwork have in the future of dentistry? After the money incentives which make Poorwork dentistry so attractive have been removed, he will eventually change his ways or simply fade away. The unit-fee system has supplied the greatest incentive to do poor work. The abolition of that system, and the adoption of more rational criteria for compensating dentists, such as the time-knowledge-experience criterion, will remove the motivation for sloppy dentistry. Of course, Dr. Poorwork may still be a problem for some time after the change to a new system of fees. After many years of utilizing the easiest, quickest, and sloppiest treatment methods, he may find it difficult to change his ways, despite the fact that poor work will no longer pay extra dividends.

But the system will breed no new Poorworks, and if old Dr. Poorwork joins a group, the group discipline will tend to keep him in line and to upgrade his work. If this did not work, then Poorwork, who after all is an experienced dentist, could be used in a capacity which would make use of his experience and ability, such as it is, and be paid accordingly. Such treatment might give him strong incentive to improve his methods. If he remains in private practice, his patients would be informed, via the enlarged program of dental education, of the nature of the treatment they have recieved from him over the years. The pressure generated by this public knowledge would give him another kind of incentive to upgrade his standards. Since many dentists would no doubt choose to remain in individual private practice and would not adopt a time-based fee system, staying with the unit fee instead, the public, now informed in the ways of dentistry by the national education program, could make an informed choice of the type of dental care it was to receive.

A particularly ticklish dimension of the problem of economics will be to determine at what levels to set fees under a time-based system. Here we raise the questions (1) How much is a dentist worth and, (2) Who is going to determine this? As to the problem of who should be qualified to set the level of fees, I say that in the long run it should be the public, the consumer, the *informed* dental consumer. Dentists can make a lot of money indeed. I know of some dentists whose yearly income from dentistry alone, under the unit-fee system, is in six figures. One Poorwork I know is in a seventy-five-per-cent tax bracket. Are these dentists worth their large incomes? I believe an *informed* public should decide, just as an informed consumer decides whether any item he wishes to purchase is worth the price. After the general public and its various group representatives insurance companies and so forth become well informed about dentistry, the fees can be established by direct negotiation with the principals themselves or with their representatives. I think the problem will work itself out, though no doubt with a good deal of turmoil, so that we will at last arrive at a rational fee system that will encourage quality dentistry and still maintain the necessary degree of professional freedom.

24

How to Avoid
Dr. Poorwork

At this point, the concerned reader will be asking himself what steps he should take to protect his oral health and to insure that the dental work he receives is of good quality. Sad to say, there is no foolproof method of obtaining good care. However there are some steps a patient can take that will increase his chances of finding a good dentist.

A reading of this book will have supplied some relevant criteria for the evaluation of a dentist's services. Appearance of the office, luxury of appointments, elegance of furnishings: these are not relevant considerations. What counts is the nature of the *service* to be provided. A person must feel that his dentist's major concern is to prevent the loss of teeth and maintain oral health.

The best way to find a good dentist is to call a local dental school and ask for the name of a faculty member

who has a practice in a convenient location. If there is
no dental school in your community, and a choice of
dentists is possible, try to interview some patients of
each dentist. Be on guard against the patient who is
enthusiastic about the painless extractions he receives.
Why is his dentist so practiced in pulling rather than
saving teeth? Make sure that the dentist schedules
patients for a specific time and then allots sufficient
time for proper treatment. And be wary of the "factory-
style" office and the overcrowded waiting room.

After you select a dentist, the preliminary dental
examination can give important insight into the quality
of care the patient can expect to receive. The examination must be thorough, and the subsequent presentation to the patient of the existing oral condition and the
treatment plan must be clear and comprehensive. (See
chapter on the Dental Examination.) The explanation
of the oral condition and the prescription for treatment
should be consistent with the principles elaborated in
this book. If the prescribed work seems unnecessarily
complex, the patient would do well to consult with
another dentist. In some cities there may be an opportunity to receive an examination and diagnosis at the
clinic of a dental school, which would be an excellent
way to receive a confirmatory diagnosis. The first
dentist, if honest, will never object to this, and will
likely welcome the opportunity to have the patient's
doubts relieved. As treatment progresses, the patient
should receive full explanations of the various phases
of the work as it is performed. It may also be helpful,
when a new phase of treatment is planned, to review the
material in this book dealing with that subject. If during the course of treatment the patient becomes aware
that too little time is being spent on restorations, that
the dentist is rushed, that periodontal work is done
hastily if at all, that the dentist is not averse to extracting teeth as a solution to difficult problems, and

that reasonable explanations of these things are not forthcoming, then it may be time to consider a change of dentist.

A person seeking dental treatment for himself and, perhaps, for his family may wish to try a novel approach which might be more effective than other methods in securing good dental services, particularly in a neighborhood where good dentistry is difficult to find. This approach involves dealing with the dentist in a manner which would eliminate the unit-fee scale, with its attendant disadvantages, so often remarked upon in this book. If the patient can arrange that routine work, excluding major prosthetic restorations, be paid for *by the hour*, he may find that he has provided a most effective incentive for good dentistry. If the dentist arranges a specific appointment, for a specific period of time, at a specific time-based fee, all of the economic factors which produce Poorwork dentistry are eliminated, and the patient stands the very best chance of receiving good work. When he is paid for a specific time period, the dentist is freed of the pressure of other patients breathing down his neck, since his time has already been assigned to the present patient. If it should develop that a filling takes much longer to complete properly, the dentist who is paid for his time will not be tempted to do a hasty and poor job, as he might were he being paid for the filling. When a difficult problem arises he will not begrudge the extra time needed for its ideal solution. On the other hand, if the dentist has some simple and easy fillings to do, he will do them properly with dispatch and at a saving to the patient. In short, the intelligent patient who deals with his dentist on a time basis is likely to enjoy superior dental care and to save money in the long run.

But it may be difficult to find a dentist willing to treat you on a time basis. My suggestion is to keep trying. If you are at last successful, your dentist is likely to be a good and understanding person and your dental health will reap the benefits.

But you still may not succeed in finding such a dentist. The idea of a time-based fee, while certainly not new, may prove to be too novel for the dentists you discuss it with. It would not be acceptable at all to Dr. Poorwork, because it would eliminate most of his opportunities for easy profit. This is too bad, because even Poorwork would find some reason to try to do good work if he were compensated on a time basis.

Summary of Things to Watch For

1. Careful examination
2. Full explanation of diagnosis and treatment plan
3. Periodontal work (gums) must not be neglected
4. Every effort should be made to avoid extractions
5. Patient should sense that the dentist is interested, is spending time, and is concentrating on the treatment
6. When treatment is finished, the mouth should feel comfortable and be functioning well; the bite should feel good and the gums should not bleed
7. If, in the months and years subsequent to treatment, fillings fall out, the gums bleed frequently or heavily, pain is common and extractions suggested, it is time to seek another dentist
8. Finally, as treatment progresses, the patient should refer to the relevant chapters in this book. If the treatment received is not consistent with the material found in these pages, a clear and convincing explanation by the dentist is in order.

25

Medicaid and Other Insurance Programs

Perhaps the major reason for the lack of progress in the development of functional dental insurance programs is the overwhelming dental need of the population. It has been estimated that only about twenty per cent of the population receives adequate dental care, and even this low figure assumes Poorwork dentistry to be adequate. Clearly, the dentally neglected and the victims of Dr. Poorwork represent an enormous backlog of dental need. Because of this backlog, it becomes almost impossibly difficult to make a close calculation of what dental-insurance premiums should be in a new program. For example, one cannot find the costs of treatment under a projected insurance program by taking present per-capita expenditures and multiplying by the number of expected participants, as is done in medicine. A person who is newly covered by medical insurance does not rush out to have his appendix re-

271

moved, or to have brain surgery; he waits until he has medical need. Only then will he cash in on his insurance. But in the case of dental insurance, the need is already there, and it is a need of a serious kind for a high percentage of the American population. The reason this need has not already been attended to is that it has not represented a threat to life, but only to dental health. But once the need is covered by insurance, watch out! The demand will be enormous.

Now that some labor contracts are beginning to include dental insurance, dentists are seeing many newly insured people who are having expensive work done that had been put off for years. A premium set at, say, fifty dollars a year, will not cover the costs of a new dental-insurance program if most of the subscribers already carry around a dental need that will cost many hundreds of dollars to correct. This has been the depressing experience of most dental insurance plans, and it has resulted in either the demise or radical alteration of dental insurance plans to date; the alterations are usually the exclusion of expensive work from the coverage.

Medicaid is a large-scale, government-sponsored program through which a participating state pays the practitioner for work performed for certain people deemed "medically indigent." Funds for this program come from Federal and state and local sources, though the pattern may vary somewhat from state to state, and each state has its own criteria of just what it is that constitutes medical indigence. New York State has gone so far as to set up special eligibility requirements for licensed dentists who wish to participate in the program. The profession has bitterly opposed these requirements; it feels that all properly licensed dentists should be allowed to treat Medicaid patients. Payments are made to the practitioner according to a set unit-fee scale. A dental Medicaid program based on the unit-fee system has a serious drawback in that reasonable fees cannot be maintained in the face of widespread low-quality work. The history of dentistry under Britain's national health service gives a good example of this. There were two classes of dentists working in England; those who were university trained, and those who learned the profession in apprentice fashion. The latter were known as blood-and-vulcanite dentists, because their approach to dentistry was to extract teeth and make full dentures. (Vulcanite is a material formerly used in the making of dentures.) After the national health service set up a unit-fee system, the blood-and-vulcanite dentists cleaned up. They didn't bother with the less profitable service of *fixing* teeth. When it became evident how much these people were making, the bureaucracy's answer to the situation was characteristic: Reduce the fees! And so the trained, conscientious dentists, already hard-pressed by the low hourly earnings afforded by fillings, now found fees so low that good work might be done only at a loss. Thus, under economic pressure, the methods of the blood-and-vulcanite dentists were widely adopted, with the result the English now have the highest incidence of false teeth in the world. Despite the generally rising cost of living, some twenty years after the beginnings of the national health service dental fees were actually lower than when the program was begun! Very recently the New York State Medicaid administration announced a reduction in certain allowable fees. Could this be the beginning, for us, of what has already happened in Britain? The tendency of the last two years seems to show that fees will be reduced to the point where only Poorwork dentistry is possible.

Although hasty, shoddy work that brings in more money under the unit-fee system is the most common abuse of the Medicaid program, certain other abuses may seem even more distasteful: unnecessary procedures, claiming previous work as one's own, asking payment for work that was not done, prescribing high-profit work in place of more-needed, low-profit work, and completely falsifying claim forms. One who scans this list of abuses might consider it unlikely that professional men would stoop so low. Incredibly evil as these abuses seem, I consider that inferior service is at least as reprehensible as any of them. A dentist who sticks in a shoddy filling is as immoral as another dentist who fakes a patient's record on a Medicaid form.

I recently complained to a dentist about the dreadful work being done under Medicaid, and about the profiteering. "Sure there is terrible work being done," he said, "and certainly there are abuses. But the program is a good thing. Remember, *people are having dental work done who otherwise would never be able to do so.*" This is the old theory, that bad work is better than none, and that it's better to give the poor something than nothing. I find this totally unacceptable.

Bad work is not better than no work at all. Bad work falls apart in a few years, and it usually leaves the patient much worse off than he was initially. After the bad work has come apart, the patient needs more complex and more expensive restorations. It is in this way that bad work usually multiplies by many times the eventual cost of treatment. But what is most scandalous is that Medicaid pays the dentist enough to do *good work*—work which will restore the mouth to health and comfort and that will preserve the teeth for long years of service. To produce poor work under such circumstances is disgraceful.

In order to make thousands of dollars each month from Medicaid *in his spare time* (since such work is presumably in addition to one's regular practice) Dr. Poorwork has had to outdo even himself in the production of hasty, poor-quality work. He has been doing this by concentrating on hurry-up fillings, extractions, and high-profit partial dentures. The figures show that children did not get as much care as they should have in the first year of Medicaid. It is hard to work on children, and they are not as profitable as adults. You can't make partial dentures for children. I suggest that it was Dr. Poorwork's reluctance to work on children, under these circumstances, which explains their neglect. These considerations do not cast a flattering light on organized dentistry, which has for too long defended Dr. Poorwork's right to practice dentistry in whatever manner he pleases.

Published statistics on Medicaid add some interesting sidelights to the above discussion. In New York City alone, $62,284,000 was expended for dentistry during the year ending August 15, 1968. This is an average of $12,261 for each participating dentist. Payments to dentists exceeded payments to physicians. At the height of the program, before the state-mandated cutbacks on patient eligibility took place, New York City dentists were receiving some ten million dollars monthly for Medicaid services. In the two-week period ending August 1, 1968, after the state cutbacks, but before their effects were felt locally, some four-and-a-half million dollars was paid to three thousand dentists in the city; that is an *average* of fifteen hundred dollars per dentist for the two weeks.

In interpreting these figures it should be borne in mind that many dentists who are represented in the figures do not have a high proportion of Medicaid patients in their practice. My own practice, for example, showed Medicaid payments of less than twelve hundred dollars for the year ending August 15, 1968; this is one-tenth the city average of over twelve thousand dollars. If many dentists receive much less than the average, then there are others who receive much more. It is safe to say, then, that many dentists received *much* more than $12,621 from the Medicaid program during the year. And if for two weeks in August the *average* dentist was paid fifteen hundred dollars, we can assume that many dentists received much more than that average. We must remember that these dentists had *no* Medicaid in their practices until recently, and that nearly all have their regular practices to keep up with. In most cases, therefore, the Medicaid payments are for only a portion of the dentist's working time. Such considerations lead one to appreciate what an enormous impact this program has had on the income of even the average dentist. It is widely known that some dentists are making enormous sums from the Medicaid program, sums so high that one must wonder just how it is possible for them to turn out so much work, and what kind of work it must be. The Medicaid administrators have recently been wondering about these same things.

One of the terrifying aspects of the Medicaid program as it is now set up in New York, for example, is that it is serving as a spawning ground for more Poorworks. Recent graduates, fresh from dental school or internship, have been attracted by the prospects for lucrative employment in one of the many factory-style practices that have been set up to exploit the Medicaid program. These practices emphasize hasty, careless work. They demand that their dentist-employees produce massive quantities of dental work without regard to its quality. With such an initiation into dental practice, and swayed by the high financial rewards of such practice, these recent graduates may quickly become confirmed Poorworks. If this happens, they will plague the profession for the rest of their lives. Thus, in this respect, Medicaid may turn out to have a lasting detrimental effect on the quality of dental practice.

In New York State, the Medicaid administrators recognize the possibility of such abuses and have set up certain well-intentioned, though feeble safeguards against them. There is, for example, a board of examining dentists to whom practitioners must submit a detailed report of work performed, plus X-rays when requested. Certain types of work require prior approval by the examining dentists; in such cases the Medicaid board, after studying X-rays submitted by the dentist, decides whether or not to allow the dentist to proceed with the restoration. In effect, this absentee board, that never sees the patient, decides whether or not the work may be done. Of course it is absurd to pass on a diagnosis and a complex restoration without ever looking at the patient, and the dentists on the board must know it. Obviously, this restraint on the practitioner has been set up only because the Medicaid administration *does not trust* the dentist, and therefore wants some check, however feeble, on his work. Have the Medicaid administrators reason to distrust the dentist? I think so. I believe they are aware of the prevalence of Poorworkism, and that the requirements for prior authorization are the result.

As one might expect, organized dentistry wants the removal of all requirements for prior authorization. The implication of the requirements—that the dentist might prescribe something not needed—is scarcely flattering, and it does not fit in with organized dentistry's party line, that all dentists are good and do good work and that their performance must not be questioned. In addition, there is the legitimate complaint that the competent and honest dentist is better qualified to prescribe than an examining board which never even looks at the patient. There is no doubt that, if all dentists suddenly became honest and conscientious, the Medicaid board would only need to set down certain guidelines for treatment. Then the honest practitioners would follow the guidelines, the requirement of prior approvals would be abandoned, and the program would operate much more smoothly.

The prior-approval regulations represent one attempt by the people running Medicaid to control the Poorworks and thus to assure good dentistry. Another attempt to upgrade the care, by eliminating the Poorworks, has been the controversial continuing-education requirement. In New York it is now mandatory that dentists participating in the Medicaid program give evidence of their continued participation in dental education. They must be either on a hospital staff or enrolled in postgraduate dental courses. Dentists taking courses must take seventy-five hours over a three-year period, including both formal courses and attendance at lectures and meetings. In the diplomatic language of a Medicaid official speaking to a dental group, such requirements are aimed at "the small minority of dentists who have not kept up with advances in the profession." He continued by saying that many of "these men" had furnished a large portion of the dental services for welfare patients before Medicaid, and that their standards were low. In other words he was telling the dental group that the bad dentists were "some other guys." But if this were the case the universal requirement need not have been adopted. For "the small minority of dentists" read "the Dr. Poorworks," who, for all we know, may be anything but a small minority.

But for all we may sympathize with the intent of the continuing-education requirement, it cannot work for dentistry. In medicine it is true that a physician not hospital-connected is seriously hampered in his ability to practice; but just about every physician in New York City, for example, is connected with a hospital and thus meets the requirement for continuing education. But in dentistry, no amount of formal courses will induce Dr. Poorwork to take the additional time necessary to fill a tooth properly. He attends many lectures as it is, and he enjoys them. But he knows that if he took more time to fill a tooth his income would decline, and that is all he cares to know. It is not very likely that while attending a postgraduate course he will suddenly become inspired to remove active decay from a tooth before filling it. He already knows the right way to fill a tooth and that it is important to do it properly. It's just that, in his view, money is even more important. The only way Dr. Poorwork will mend his ways is if it becomes economically attractive for him to do so. This will happen only if good work becomes more lucrative than poor work. No amount of continuing education will change his ways, and the Medicaid continuing-education requirement as it stands is therefore simply ludicrous.

A laughable aspect of the continuing-education requirement is that it can be entirely satisfied by courses in practice management! Thus Dr. Poorwork can take a few occasional weekends off and attend some of the many practice-management seminars which are held aboard cruise ships and in such dentally significant places as Miami, Puerto Rico, Hawaii, Aruba, Portugal, and so on. After being professionally elevated by a tax-deductible weekend discussing practice management on the beaches and in the casinos of these resorts, Dr. Poorwork can return to his profitable work of mutilating mouths. And the New York State Department of Health will show its appreciation of these educational efforts by granting him continued eligibility to render his selfless attentions to the medically indigent.

It would be more sensible to make prospective patients take courses in dentistry. This suggestion is not entirely facetious; the Medicaid patient, having learned something of dentistry through formal courses, would not stand for Dr. Poorwork's brand of care. The patient's rejection of Poorwork methods, and his insistence upon quality dentistry, would do more to upgrade Medicaid practice than any courses Poorwork might take.

Another measure that the Medicaid administrators might consider, in their efforts to improve the dentistry under the program, would be to set up a scale of standards for the quality of treatment, apply these standards to the output of the various dentists, and *periodically publicize the results*. A dentist's practice might be studied as to the number of teeth lost by his patients over a period of time, the number of restoration failures, "broken" fillings, teeth "gone bad," and so forth. I am satisfied that the publication of such data, naming names, would provide much more incentive for good dentistry than the irrelevant continuing-education requirement. Of course, if all dentists involved in public programs were subject to publishable quality evaluations, then each dental treatment would become an item in a competitive examination. There is nothing wrong with this; every bit of dentistry done by a dentist should test the dentist to do his very best. Aiming for anything less than the best result is reprehensible, and the state has every right to reject inferior treatment in state-supported programs. Nor would publication of the quality levels of dentists cause patients to flock to one particular man, the one with the highest marks, because all trained, conscientious dentists would fare almost equally well in these competitions, and all should be able to achieve excellent ratings. The steady competition of such evaluations would supply a lasting incentive to good dentistry.

A useful parallel measure would be to test and grade patients participating in public programs in such matters as oral hygiene and the keeping of appointments, for example. Patients who waste the dentist's time by missing appointments and who waste his skill by neglecting oral hygiene might have their eligibility suspended until they can show improvement.

Now that the Medicaid statistics are beginning to cast a little light on the activities of Dr. Poorwork, organized dentistry must, and without delay, take steps to eliminate Poorworkism. The alternative will be to sit back and let government do the job. As we have seen, the Medicaid people are already making efforts to control the quality of the dentistry they are purchasing. Recently there has been talk on official levels of prosecuting cases of suspected fraud, withholding payment for defective services, and suspending practitioners from the program. A peer review committee has also been under consideration. In the early stages of the program, as many as thirty per cent of treatment plans submitted to Medicaid had to be revised by the Medicaid staff dentists. A desire to upgrade the projected treatment was given as a major reason for the need of revision. On the subject of "substandard services," a Medicaid official recently said, "It's really not a question of the dentist's ability, but of his conscience and the pressures of the moment." This point is central to my main point in this book: All duly licensed dentists are capable of performing good work, but "the pressures of the moment," i.e., the desire to make money, and lack of conscience, result in poor work by too many dentists.

I will finish with some ominous words by a high

Medicaid official, referring to a legal action concerning the controversial continuing-education requirement: "This action should . . . test the prerogative of government or perhaps any purchaser of health services to set the qualifications of its professional provider panels." The signs are clear. If organized dentistry continues to refuse to police itself, then government will certainly do the policing for it.

26

New Directions and Solutions

The most important problem in dentistry today is the massive dental need of the population. It is believed, for example, that only twenty per cent of the population receives adequate dental care; the percentage must be a good deal lower when we subtract the victims of Dr. Poorwork. This will not do for a prosperous, progressive country with humane ideals. The country has a dental problem of its own, and it is this problem that sets the stage for the drama about to be enacted within the dental profession.

It has become urgent that dentistry make a number of decisions about its future, but the questions are not being formulated rapidly enough, and the answers are slow in coming. Shall we plan to serve more people, and eventually all the people, or shall we cater mainly to the few, as at present? Shall we be content with security

283

and pride of accomplishment in our work, or shall we scheme to make more wealth for ourselves?

The choice may not be so easy. If organized dentistry plans mostly for itself, as it has in the past, it should not be surprised when it comes into conflict with a nation that must increasingly plan for *it*self. Such a head-on collision can have only one result: Dental practice will be changed to fit the needs and ideas of people outside the profession. If, on the other hand, dentists decide to devote themselves increasingly to the ideal of service, there is the possibility that the means by which they choose to do so will be the wrong ones. In either case, the result might be no better, or possibly even worse, than what we have now: In the end we might find many more people receiving the "benefits" of shoddy dentistry, while fewer than ever received proper care.

The time for decision is now and over the next very few years. One way or another, dentists will have to make dental care available to much more of the population. This central challenge breaks down into the several subordinate challenges of quality, public education, economics, trained personnel, facilities, and distribution.

Traditionally, the dentist has been a rugged individualist, working for the most part by himself in his own private office. His freedom, professional as well as personal, was complete. In dealing with his patients he selected his own treatment options, limited perhaps only by the patient's ability to pay for expensive treatment; he was otherwise free to do as he saw fit. If in his judgment a certain method of treatment was best for the patient, he did not have to submit his opinions to a bureaucratic panel for approval; he just went ahead and treated the patient according to his own lights. He was the only and final authority on the soundness and appropriateness of his treatment. His freedom extended in other directions: He was his own boss; he could schedule patients as he wished, take vacations as he wished, work hard or leisurely as he wished. More so than the great majority of people, the dentist was his own man, accountable only to himself. Although dentistry can be exhausting and aggravating, it is this freedom which, added to accomplishment, supplied the greatest gratification to most practitioners. It is not surprising, then, that dentists have resisted changes that might tend to diminish these freedoms.

But the fact is that our rugged-individualist dentist has not done the job; he simply has failed to meet the need for adequate dental care, though it hasn't been entirely his fault. The idea that universal medical and dental care are a citizen's right has only recently been developed. Indeed, this notion still sounds downright revolutionary to some, who bitterly resist it. But the idea is here to stay and, as society further broadens the concept of universal health care, the demand for care will increase many fold. The rugged-individualist dentist is not going to be able to supply the need, and the traditional concept of private dental practice must, with some nostalgic regrets, give way to other forms of practice.

Speculation concerning these new forms must take into account the problems listed above, of quality, public education, economics, facilities, trained personnel, and distribution. A number of the ideas for the improvement of dental service that have been advanced have given insufficient weight to the need to solve one or more of these basic problems. Some proposed programs scarcely depart from tradition, while others would radically alter the character and structure of dentistry as a profession. Any suggested alternatives to traditional practice must be critically examined to determine whether they in fact offer a real improvement over traditional concepts, or merely offer change for the sake of change. In this situation, all that is wholly clear are the problems listed above, and that some sort of change is inevitable.

The individual private practice, while offering many attractions and advantages, has within its structure a great many disadvantages, both professional and personal, both to the dentist and to his patients. The dentist has found it difficult to take vacations, which might leave his practice uncovered; provisions for emergency treatment in his absence have been awkward. There has been little day-to-day opportunity for the interchange of professional ideas. Under such conditions it is possible even for the conscientious dentist to become professionally stale and to lapse, almost unthinkingly, into inferior ways of working.

The tendency of the lone private practitioner to go his own way may in the long run adversely affect the quality of his output and the extent of his continued interest. Both the practitioner and his patients might suffer for it, the practitioner finding his work less challenging and too routine, and the patients perhaps receiving imperfect care.

Since this may happen to the most conscientious and careful of dentists, imagine what happens when Dr. Poorwork is let loose on his patients under conditions of private practice. He has always interpreted the freedom of private practice as license to do as he pleases with his patients, and he has usually pleased to do what is most profitable to himself without regard for their well-being. Insulated as he has been by the protection and privileges of his private practice, Dr. Poorwork has engendered abuses so monstrous that they now represent the most immediate threat to the system of private practice. Purchasers of dentistry through group programs, including government, insurance companies, and unions, are lately becoming aware of Dr. Poorwork and his methods, and to protect themselves they are beginning to devise and set up systems of quality control which will ultimately destroy the absolute freedom dentists have enjoyed.

Private practice has also failed to come to grips with any of the other major problems of dentistry. While some dentists spend much time in the education of their patients, others do not. Even those dentists who are disposed to use their time for patient-education have not been able to reach all those people who avoid dental offices for reasons of fear, misunderstanding, lack of dental knowledge, and so on. The problem of economics has been most serious in private practice; it has prevented patients from getting needed care, made it difficult to practice good-quality dentistry in many neighborhoods, and spawned countless Poorworks. And the traditional system of private practice has not produced nearly enough dentists, trained personnel, and facilities to serve the population. Add to all this that private practice has failed to establish a rational, nation-wide distribution of dentists and facilities. Applying the criteria of these considerations, then, it seems that traditional private practice has fallen far short of society's present needs.

But tradition dies hard, particularly with the group privileged by tradition. It is understandable that dentists who have enjoyed the freedoms and advantages afforded by private practice will fight to preserve their status. But a more cogent reason is needed; private practice can no longer be defended merely on the ground that the dentist likes it. Of course, many attempts have been made to justify the cherished institution. Indeed, even to suggest alternatives has often been regarded as heresy. Private practice, it has been said, is the foundation of professional excellence and progress. Without private practice and its attendant freedoms, it has been said, the quality of care will suffer and effective research will be stifled. It is said that only the incentives offered by private practice can insure the maintenance of the highest levels of professional performance and outlook. It is also argued, and with great sincerity, that the profession, both as a discipline and as a vocation, would be degraded by any system incorporating even the possibility of bureaucratic fetters that would entangle the free spirit of practice and interfere with the doctor's right to prescribe for his patient.

So goes the party line, and it has occurred to very few to challenge it. This is the way things have always been; why should we change? But the possibility of change must be freshly evaluated when there are new factors to consider. Today we must ask whether private practice is in fact essential to the maintenance of quality in dentistry. Ask Dr. Poorwork, but when he answers just remember who he is and what he does and what institution it is that defends his right to do it in private. Ask the Medicaid and insurance officials, who are becoming acquainted with Poorwork's concept of quality in private practice. Ask the union officials responsible for purchasing dental care for their membership. Ask the patients of Dr. Poorwork, those who have awoken in time to see another dentist before losing their dental health entirely. It is the unrestricted freedoms of private practice that have allowed Dr. Poorwork to flourish, and which have actually sustained dentistry of the lowest quality. This consideration should be enough to dispose of the idea that private practice is the watchdog of high quality. Finally, ask organized dentistry, whose membership opposes the Medicaid unit-fee system in favor of "customary and reasonable fees"—a fact which obliquely suggests that differences in quality do indeed exist and should be reflected in differences in fees.

Private practice is certainly not essential to free and active research. The fact is that the fruits of serious research almost never come from the offices of private practitioners, but always from the clinics and laboratories of institutions. Although men engaged in private practice may conduct much research, invariably the useful work is organized and channeled through institutional facilities; the actual research is almost never done in the private office. And though innovations in techniques and treatments often do come from private practitioners, the correlative research is done by or at the institution.

Another sacred cow has been the doctor's "inviolate right" to prescribe treatment for his patient. Interfere with this cherished right, say the old-line theoreticians, and you strike a death blow at the very heart of professionalism. Well, I think it is high time that this concept be reexamined. This cherished, inviolate right to prescribe and perform whatever treatment one likes on one's patient is apparently conferred on the chosen man by a dental-school diploma and a state license; it is these pieces of paper which transform the man from a mortal with full responsibility for his actions to a god who is not to be questioned and who is immune from responsibility. Unfortunately this so-called right is today being grossly abused by Dr. Poorwork, who invokes it to justify his peculiar brand of shoddy dentistry, according to which his patients' dental health is at best secondary in importance to his own material advancement. Certainly the ancient right to prescribe without interference from anybody or anything is not worth the price Dr. Poorwork is forcing the country to pay for it. Some limitations must be defined and enforced. Now is the time for the profession to cut its losses. An intelligent look at the alternatives today may reduce the practitioner's loss of freedom tomorrow.

There is, indeed, one very important argument in favor of private practice that must not be overlooked. Private practice allows the patient to deal directly with his dentist on a personal basis, rather than with an impersonal panel or institution. This has been a most important advantage, and must be kept in mind when contemplating any plans for change in the structure of dental practice.

The concept of private *group* practice has been advanced as an attractive alternative to individual private practice. A group practice is a practice conducted by more than one dentist; it may mean two or five or more dentists sharing the same facilities and, to some extent, the same patients. The group-practice idea is not new; in medicine, groups have flourished for some time, and more recently dental group practices have been making headway. Group practice definitely abridges the freedom of the individual dentist, who must defer to his partner or his group.

Yet the group approach to dentistry has its own strong advantages, which deserve to be considered. The fact that there are one or more other dentists present can in itself lead to a great boost in the quality of care. The ability to consult quickly with a colleague can be very helpful and reassuring to the dentist with a difficult case. I have had experience with group practice in the Army, and with individual private practice in my own office over the past many years. As I compare the two experiences, I am convinced that under the conditions of group practice my present burdens would be eased and the resultant quality of my work improved. There are times when, under the stress of time, the practitioner has difficulty seeing what might be an obvious solution to another man, who can take a fresh and detached view of the problem.

In the Army I had just such experiences. If I was bogged down in a problem with a patient, one quick look by a colleague could often resolve the situation. And just as he helped me, so I was able to help my colleague with his problems. Many times, in my private practice, I have felt the need of a helping hand or a sympathetic word in a difficult situation. In a group, the practitioner is not alone; and this fact supplies him with practical and emotional support that enables him to do a better job. In the case of larger group practices there is the additional possibility of having specialists practicing on the same premises, with the great convenience and advantages of their expertise being readily available.

Under the conditions of group practice it may also be possible to share specialized equipment which the lone private dentist could not afford for his single practice. If the group is large enough it may be able to hire its own laboratory technician, who would be on the premises and susceptible to immediate supervision by the dentist; this would result in a great saving of time and more accurate laboratory work. Besides technicians, other auxiliary personnel might with advantage be shared by the group: hygienists, nurses, and secretaries, for example. Patient-education facilities such as consulting rooms, projection and demonstration equipment, and exhibits might be supported by a group. Such facilities are beyond the means of most individual practitioners. A group practice can realize many economies in shared overhead, including rent, equipment, maintenance, record-keeping, and personnel. These economies can be translated into some of the improved facilities mentioned above.

The dentist in a group can plan a needed vacation without worrying about leaving his practice unattended; if a patient needs emergency attention in his absence, a colleague in the same office, who knows the patient and who has access to the records and history of the case, will be available to handle the situation. Perhaps most important of all, the presence of each dentist's colleagues in a well-run group practice with high ideals will continually stimulate him to do his best, and the entire group will tend to remain alert and up-to-date. It is understandable that a dentist in a group practice would be embarrassed to have a substandard piece of work reviewed by a colleague. When the responsibility of treatment is thus shared by conscientious dentists, the quality of treatment will tend to rise to the highest possible level. This is the desirable situation dentistry must aim for, and it is in striking contrast to the incentives generated in private practice by the unit-fee system and Poorwork competition.

Group practice also provides the flexibility in personnel, equipment, and facilities to utilize the most modern concepts of practice. Time and motion studies in dentistry have been made with a view to making the performance of dental procedures more efficient. These studies have led to newly designed equipment and new procedures such as the four-handed and quadrant concepts in which the dentist and an auxiliary work on the patient simultaneously. The studies point the way to more efficient utilization of the dentist's time and to the speeding up of quality dentistry.

A further, possibly great advantage of the group-practice idea is that a group might be designed to include one or more dentists having specialized knowl-lege and experience. The advantage of such a set-up becomes clear, for example, when one reflects that the good dentist whose practice consists mainly of people who care about their teeth is rarely required to make full dentures. The good dentists of my acquaintance make very few dentures, and actually have had relatively little clinical experience with denture patients. This is because their patients do not lose their teeth, and the number of transient, toothless patients who come in is very low. It might make sense, therefore, if the designing of full dentures were set aside as a specialty area. At the very least it might be a good idea to have a specialist to supervise denture work, and at the same time train those he is supervising. (Of course, Dr. Poorwork has had much more experience with dentures than the good dentist has. Assuming that Poorwork takes the time to do his denture work carefully, which he probably does not, he might well be better at dentures than most good dentists are.)

But there are definite drawbacks to the group-practice idea. One has already been mentioned, that of a certain loss of freedom. In a group, the dentist would lose his former ability to schedule as he pleased and to treat as he pleased. The latter is no drawback; the freedom to treat as one pleases has been remarkable only for its abuse. No dentist should accept less than his best effort, and it is precisely each man's best that the good group practice will demand. As for scheduling, an intelligent group will well understand the physical demands of dentistry and will arrange for sufficient flexibility in scheduling to accommodate each dentist's need for an occasional breather. Nevertheless, some of the dentist's prior freedom in this respect will be lost.

Whenever efficiency is overemphasized there is a clear danger that quality will suffer and that the patient will be forgotten. While four-handed and quadrant methods can indeed increase efficiency, they cannot radically raise the output of quality dentistry. The patient is not a workbench, but a human being; dentistry must not overlook his humanity for the sake of efficiency. It takes a certain irreducible amount of time to fit a crown, to cement an inlay, to remove deep decay, or to plug, condense, and carve a silver filling. These and many other critical procedures can only be speeded up at the expense of adequate results. The dentist or group concentrating on efficiency may occasionally be tempted to cut corners in order to meet optimistic schedules. If this happens, it will just be Poorwork dentistry all over again. In fact, the biggest potential problem in the group-practice idea is the threat of Dr. Poorwork. A group practice set up with Poorwork economic motives and Poorwork service ideals will be just that much more efficient in destroying its patients' dental health. Alas, many group practices today are just factories supplying Poorwork dentistry. Many of these factories have been set up to take advantage of Medicaid and to exploit the poor; some of these practices have recently been making headlines.

Even if a group establishes and maintains high standards of practice, there is always the latent danger that the treatment may become too efficiently organized, too routinized, and too impersonal. Most patients want to have a personal relationship with their doctor, and many groups have achieved this goal by having each patient cared for mostly by one dentist, while at the same time encouraging him to become acquainted with the other practitioners.

There are many possible types of group dental practice. Some groups are strictly private in character, and draw their support from the general public on a private basis. Some groups have direct organizational, institutional, or government support. Others limit their patients to members of a specific organization, union, company, insurance plan, or economic group. Some limit their work to children or to the elderly.

Much of the experience with union group practices has been depressing, the allowed coverage and economic incentives being, in too many cases, such that a very poor standard of work is established. But some union group practices have shown that superior work can be achieved. Some unions, for example, have sponsored group clinic-type practices that have achieved excellent results, which should be expected if there are incentives for good dentistry, if the practice is well equipped, and if the man in charge is honest and knowledgeable. It is, I believe, the experience of the best of these union group practices that will point the way to the improved dental services of the future. Despite its potential drawbacks and disadvantages, the concept of a well-organized, high-ideal group practice is sufficiently flexible to allow for changes designed to eliminate the problems facing dentistry. Private practice does not offer this flexibility, and can never be a vehicle for the solution of today's problems, or of tomorrow's. Sooner or later, therefore, individual private practice must give way almost completely to group practice of one kind or another.

The compassionate society must make provision for the adequate dental care of its citizens, and dentistry must be set up to meet the need. This will require a many-fold increase in dental manpower and facilities. The scope of the problem is staggering. Our dental schools as they are now constituted can train but a fraction of the needed men, and our present number of dentists, even doing the best standard of work at the highest possible efficiency, is woefully inadequate to the demands of current dental need. To set up and staff only a single dental school is a tremendously difficult task; yet many schools are needed. Somehow, in any case, the job of finding the needed manpower must be done. To this end some concerned dentists are studying ideas which, by traditional standards, might be considered radical. These ideas involve changes in dental education, changes in the legal structure of dental practice, formation of new categories of dental personnel, and expansion of the activities of auxiliary personnel.

Many dentists and dental students have long considered the present dental school curricula to be oppressive and often unnecessarily irrelevant. The dental student in his first two years of study must complete essentially the same academic work as the medical student, and *in addition to this* must carry a variety of courses in dentistry. Full medical courses in Anatomy, Pathology, Histology, Physiology, Biochemistry, Bacteriology, and Pharmacology are given to aspiring dentists in addition to all their major courses in Dentistry and minor courses in Medicine. Most dentists I know believe that this heavy volume of work contributes in no way to dental education or to the dentist's ability to perform his work. It has been proposed that these courses be sensibly abridged for dental students, so that the course could be reduced to three years, with emphasis on clinical work. This would help to turn out more fully trained dentists with present school facilities.

A more radical suggestion for dealing with the shortage of dentists is the proposal that the laws be changed to allow some significant phases of dental work to be done by personnel other than dentists. I, for one, am convinced that trained auxiliary personnel must play an important role in the future of dentistry. People can be trained in a relatively short time to perform many of the less complex dental procedures. Among several studies of the utilization of personnel other than dentists to perform dental work, one showed that fillings done by trained non-dentists compared well, in terms of quality, to fillings done by experienced dentists; another showed that work done by non-dentists with limited training was ofter *superior* to work done by dental students. It does seem logical that personnel trained to do general dental procedures should be utilized once they have satisfactorily demonstrated their capability. Such auxiliary practitioners would not, of course, be qualified to evaluate cases and prescribe treatment. These decisions would always be in the province of the fully trained dentist; so would many of the more difficult dental procedures.

The use of such trained auxiliaries, in a group practice or clinic set-up, under close supervision by a fully qualified dentist who prescribes, checks on all work, and assists in difficult procedures, would seem to be a rational possibility for the future. Such a set-up might increase the output of quality dentistry, per dentist, by as much as five times. The utilization of auxiliaries will require some changes in law and attitude. Auxiliaries might be separated into different legal categories, according to training and experience, and allowed to perform different types of work accordingly. Auxiliaries could be used to take X-rays, clean teeth, fill teeth, do more complex restorations, and do periodontal scalings, according to their legal classification. In such a framework, the attending dentists might consider the teaching of auxiliary personnel to be part of their function. Indeed, any solution to the dental manpower problem must attempt to use a high percentage of dentists as teachers, at least on a part-time basis.

The concept of auxiliaries and revised standards of training can even be applied to specialties. Let us consider orthodontia, for example. The orthodontist limits his practice to a severely restricted area of dental practice in which he uses very little of his general dental and medical training. Specialized institutions could be set up to train orthodontic auxiliary personnel and even orthodontists. By concentrating on orthodontic training, the curriculum could shorten considerably the time needed to produce orthodontically trained personnel. In practice, auxiliaries could take impressions, construct, fit, and cement bands, and make minor adjustments, all the while receiving training, apprentice-fashion, from the attending orthodontists. The latter would diagnose, plan treatment, supervise, make major adjustments, and train auxiliaries and future orthodontists. In this way the supply of orthodontically trained personnel would be quickly increased, and orthodontic fees, which are now extraordinarily high for a relatively uncomplicated specialty, could be brought down to reasonable levels.

The training of these auxiliaries might be accomplished through a combination of formal courses and carefully supervised apprenticeship programs to be conducted in schools and clinics. Present facilities are inadequate; additional schools, training centers, and clinics will have to be provided. Group practices and clinics can be used both for dispensing dental services and for training of auxiliaries. These group practices and clinics might be financed by government programs, union or company organizations, or insurance programs. It begins to seem that the only realistic hope for the financing of new dental schools lies in the direction of government support; if the new projected dental schools were training centers for auxiliaries as well as for dentists, it might be more logical for government to lend its support. The possibilities are many, but the central fact remains that we still need many more schools, training centers, offices, and clinics if we are to begin to make an intelligent effort to meet the country's dental need.

The expansion of facilities for the training of personnel should be accompanied by greater efforts to educate the public in the ways of dental health. A patient with a reasonable understanding of dentistry and oral health is not likely to tolerate the sloppy care of Dr. Poorwork; broad-gauge dental education would provide a strong incentive for Dr. Poorwork to change his ways. An informed public may be the strongest safeguard against poor dentistry.

A study of the distribution of dentists reveals that certain areas are relatively saturated with dentists, while people in other areas have a hard time finding anybody to care for their teeth. It is natural for a professional man to settle where he thinks he can prosper and live well; that is why the affluent urban areas have the greatest concentration of dentists relative to population. To achieve a more reasonable distribution of dental personnel and facilities it will be necessary to supply strong incentives to attract trained people to relatively unattractive areas. Professionally, the incentives already exist. The opportunity to bring quality care to a hitherto neglected area will be most attractive to many young men. But the economic incentives must also be there, and today the dentist who goes to a neglected area to help the people there usually has to accept a meager income, even after his practice is established. Government sponsorship of practices and clinics in these areas may be the only feasible solution to the maldistribution of dental talent. In a free society we cannot order trained personnel to practice in unattractive areas, but we can learn to provide incentives strong enough to make such practice attractive.

The attempt to meet the great dental need of the country must be ambitious and will be costly, but not so costly that the country cannot afford it. The possible methods of financing a large dental program are many, and all deserve consideration. Perhaps the easiest way out is to expect the government to take control of the whole program; this would involve a government takeover of the profession, or socialized dentistry, to put it another way.

But the socialization of the profession would cause so great an upheaval that many people who today enjoy good dentistry would no longer be able to secure effective dental care, and the general quality of the work of many of even the best dentists might decline. Even if it were possible to effect the transition without chaos, the newly socialized profession would be subject to the same ills that afflict all bureaucratic organizations. The drawbacks are well known: the possibility of corruption, the limitations on the action of the individual (and the corresponding loss of initiative), the sense of helplessness caused by the incompetence of a bureaucratic supervisory appointee, the intrusion of politics and the spoils system, the fear of innovation, and the difficulty in getting quick decisions on matters needing approval. These customarily attributed traits of bureaucracy scarcely suggest a mechanism designed to meet the country's dental need, now or in the future. Nor has the experience of other countries with nationalized dentistry been heartening. The level of dental care in England is bad, according to what I have been told and the little I have seen of it. My own greatest horror of bureaucratic dentistry is that when I report to the government office for work the first day, I find that my immediate supervisor is none other than Dr. Poorwork. And don't think it couldn't happen.

Suppose, however, that dentistry does indeed solve all its problems. What might the patient then expect of dentistry? What will be the experience of a patient seeking dental care? Here follows a possible answer, optimistically projected into the very near future.

Patient A is a man who has been receiving good-quality regular dental care from a group practice. He has made an appointment for his routine check-up. He appears at the appointed time and presents himself to the receptionist, who directs him to one of the examining rooms, where he receives a clinical oral examination and has his history brought up to date by the dentist who has been mainly responsible for his care. His dentist decides that it is time for an X-ray examination and that the patient also needs a routine scaling. The patient now goes to the X-ray room, where the type of X-ray series ordered by the dentist is taken by a licensed auxiliary. At the patient's next appointment he is seated in a treatment room, where the routine scaling is done by an auxiliary. The same dentist comes in several times during the procedure to supervise and perhaps modify treatment according to the results of the X-rays. At the end of the scaling the patient is fully examined by his dentist. The scaling is checked and, if necessary, completed by the dentist, the X-rays are analyzed and compared with the clinical appearance of the mouth, and the patient's oral hygiene is checked and commented upon. The patient, who does not need further work, is dismissed until his next recall examination. On the way out he stops at the desk and is put down for recall in six months, or whatever the dentist has prescribed. Financial matters are not discussed; we assume this patient is covered by one of the many private, public, or organizational prepayment plans.

Mr. B is a regular patient who has phoned in to describe a problem; he is in pain. This is indeed rather unusual for steady patients of this group practice, who receive the best of care and, as a result, rarely experience pain. Nevertheless, Mr. B has pain, and his request for treatment is honored with an immediate appointment. He is seated in the diagnostic room where his dentist, if available, or another dentist if his personal dentist is not available, conducts a preliminary examination. If it proves to be a simple matter, the dentist may correct it at once, right at the diagnostic chair. A complex problem may require X-rays and other diagnostic aids. In any case, emergency treatment will be performed as soon as possible by the dentist or qualified auxiliary with a view to relieving the pain.

Mrs. C is not a previous patient of the group, and she is also in pain. (Despite the excellence of the community dental education program, some people still wait until an episode of pain before they seek care.) After the receptionist has received the emergency patient and begun a chart, the patient goes to a diagnostic room, where a dentist undertakes to determine the immediate cause of pain. (In such patients there often are many possible sources of trouble, all needing correction, but only one of which is causing the pain.) When the source of pain is discovered, appropriate remedial measures are taken, probably by the dentist, since such situations usually require the expertise of the experienced practitioner. The dentist may use the episode as an opportunity to teach the auxiliaries.

When the pain is relieved, the patient reports to the

receptionist for an appointment for a complete examination. At this next appointment she has a full diagnostic set of X-rays taken by an auxiliary, and she meets
her own dentist at the diagnostic chair, where he performs a clinical examination, charts obvious defects
and the periodontal condition, and arranges for any
emergency procedures. Another auxiliary, this time a
hygienist, completes the visit with a lesson in oral hygiene. At the next visit the dentist reviews the X-rays,
completes the examination, establishes a plan of treatment, and, if feasible, begins the work, usually with periodontal treatment. Because the patient needs a great
amount of work, long appointments are set up, and the
restorative work is done by four-handed, quadrant
methods. Two auxiliaries of differing qualifications, one
doing the main procedures and the other assisting, perform the work under the supervision of the dentist, who
briefs the auxiliaries and then checks on various phases
of the work, in progress and at completion, and helps
them as necessary. Several such visits may be needed
for the completion of a great deal of restorative work,
which brings the patient back to good dental health.
She is now a member of the group's family of patients;
with careful oral-hygiene practice and attention to recall appointments, she may never again encounter a
serious dental problem.

Mr. D, who wishes to become a patient of the group,
makes an appointment for examination. Because of
neglect or many years of Poorwork dentistry, he requires an enormous amount of corrective work. Several
key teeth are missing, and other teeth are infected or
are in periodontal jeopardy. During the first few visits
a complete diagnosis is performed and the most urgent
emergency work is done. The patient's own dentist, in
consultation with his colleagues and the specialists of

the group, establishes an ambitious treatment plan of great complexity, calling for multiple restorations coupled with fixed and removable bridgework. During the next several visits closely supervised auxiliaries complete the periodontal work and preliminary restorations. When work on major restorations commences, the dentist is present for each critical procedure, either to do it himself or to supervise. The dentist continually reevaluates the case and changes the treatment plan whenever it seems advisable. Dental laboratory work is done by the group's own laboratory technician under the close supervision of the dentist. As the treatment nears completion, the dentist himself attends to the delicate business of fittings, adjustments, and corrections. When the case has been completed, Mr. D becomes a member of the group's family of patients, and if he is careful he can expect little trouble in the future.

Patient E's mouth has not stood up to the years of neglect and Poorwork abuse, and his few remaining teeth are not salvageable; he needs full dentures. He is assigned to the dentist with the most specialized knowledge of dentures, who takes advantage of the teaching opportunity for the regular dentists in the group.

Patient F is a child. The group may or may not have a separate section for children's dentistry. In any case, the treatment of children requires time, patience, and expertise, and in the future will be essentially the same as described in the chapter on the Care of Children's Teeth.

Here it is appropriate to summarize the problems facing dentistry, and the projected solutions to these problems. Essentially, what all the problems boil down to is *the requirement that we meet the dental need of the country.* We must catch up with the backlog of dental need and we have to keep pace with new dental need as it develops. To reach this goal, dentistry needs a great increase in effective manpower. New training facilities, revised curricula and qualification standards, and extensive use of auxiliary personnel will increase the numbers of dental personnel and will make our existing dentists more productive. Poor-quality work is a complete waste to the patient, usually increasing his dental need, and it is a complete waste of the training and time of the practitioner. Quality levels must be improved and maintained. A more sensible, modern concept of practice and a rational system of payment can create the environment and the incentives for consistently good work. The growing need of the population, owing to new cavities, and so forth, should be attacked through national programs of prevention. Public-health programs such as fluoridation should be backed up by national patient-education campaigns focusing on oral hygiene, the best of all preventives, and the preventive value of regular dental care. Finally, there should be intensified research into the poorly understood areas of caries and periodontal disease.

I believe a program such as the above makes sense, can be ultimately successful, and will cost the public less in the long run than our present inefficient and even self-defeating approach. In addition, the suggested program would at last give dentistry its first opportunity to succeed in its purpose: to maintain the teeth and the oral health of all our people.